Color Doppler of Congenital Heart Disease in the Child and Adult

---

Edited by

Achi Ludomirsky, M.D.
Fellow in Pediatric Cardiology
The Lillie Frank Abercrombie Section of Cardiology
Department of Pediatrics
Baylor College of Medicine
Houston, Texas

and

James C. Huhta, M.D.
Associate Professor of Pediatrics and Obstetrics and Gynecology
The Lillie Frank Abercrombie Section of Cardiology
Department of Pediatrics
Baylor College of Medicine;
Director of Pediatric Echocardiography
Texas Children's Hospital and Jefferson Davis Hospital
Houston, Texas

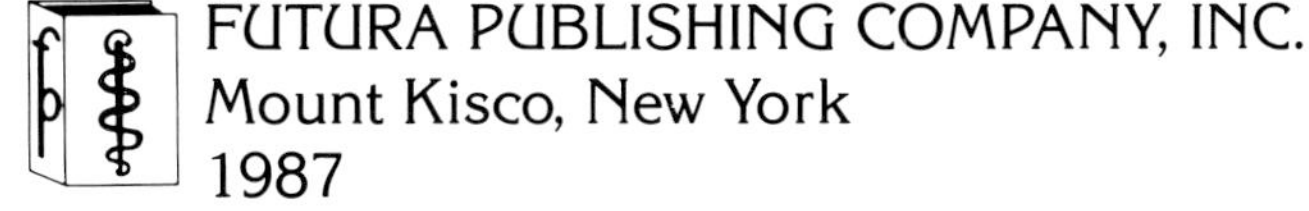

FUTURA PUBLISHING COMPANY, INC.
Mount Kisco, New York
1987

Library of Congress Cataloging-in-Publication Data

Color Doppler of congenital heart disease in the child and adult.

Includes bibliographies and index.
1. Heart—Abnormalities—Diagnosis. 2. Doppler ultrasonography. 3. Ultrasonic cardiography. 4. Pediatric cardiology. I. Ludomirsky, Achi. II. Huhta, James.
[DNLM: 1. Echocardiography—atlases. 2. Heart Defects, Congenital—diagnosis—atlases. WG 17 C7187]
RC687.C63 1987 616.1'207'543 86-46351
ISBN 0-87993-295-3

Published by
Futura Publishing Company, Inc.
295 Main Street, P.O. Box 330
Mount Kisco, New York 10549

L.C. no.: 86-46351
ISBN no.: 0-87993-295-3

Contributors

David A. Danford, M.D.
Assistant Professor of Pediatrics
The Lillie Frank Abercrombie Section of Cardiology
Department of Pediatrics
Baylor College of Medicine
Houston, Texas

Donald Hagler, M.D., F.A.C.C.
Professor of Pediatrics, Mayo Medical School
Consultant in Pediatric Cardiology
Mayo Clinic
Rochester, Minnesota

James C. Huhta, M.D., F.A.C.C.
Associate Professor of Pediatrics and Obstetrics and Gynecology
The Lillie Frank Abercrombie Section of Cardiology
Department of Pediatrics
Baylor College of Medicine
Director of Pediatric Echocardiography
Texas Children's Hospital and Jefferson Davis Hospital
Houston, Texas

Victoria E. Judd, M.D.
Assistant Professor of Pediatrics
The Lillie Frank Abercrombie Section of Cardiology
Department of Pediatrics
Baylor College of Medicine
Houston, Texas

Achi Ludomirsky, M.D.
Fellow in Pediatric Cardiology
The Lillie Frank Abercrombie Section of Cardiology
Department of Pediatrics
Baylor College of Medicine
Houston, Texas

William Robert Morrow, M.D.
Major, Assistant Chief of Cardiology
Dept of Pediatrics
Wilford Hall USAF Medical Center
at Lackland Air Force Base, Texas

Daniel J. Murphy, Jr., M.D.
Assistant Professor of Pediatrics
The Lillie Frank Abercrombie Section of Cardiology
Department of Pediatrics
Baylor College of Medicine
Houston, Texas

Foreword

During the past decade, echocardiography has matured into a powerful diagnostic tool. Today, high-resolution 2D echocardiography and Doppler echocardiographic hemodynamic evaluation can be substituted for large portions of the invasive examination. Color flow imaging is a new Doppler ultrasound technology that visualizes flow within the heart chambers and vessels. This modality can be likened to a noninvasive angiogram and is having a significant impact on the diagnosis and functional assessment of congenital heart disease. Color flow imaging and related echocardiographic technologies represent the most significant advancement in the study of congenital heart disease since the advent of cardiac catheterization, permitting anatomical, functional, hemodynamic, and new "angiographic" assessment. Presently, the logical and expeditious management of congenital heart disease patients mandates the routine use of noninvasive echocardiography and Doppler. With color flow mapping, blood flow within the heart and vessels can also be visualized and imparts an "angiographic" capability to a comprehensive examination. Today, a fully equipped echo/Doppler laboratory, capable of performing anatomical and functional assessment may be more properly termed an "Ultrasound Imaging and Hemodynamic Laboratory."

Doctors Ludomirsky and Huhta have put together an impressive compendium of color flow Doppler examinations of congenital heart disease in both children and adults. They present their experience using multiple commercially available color flow imaging instruments and present examples of most forms of congenital heart disease. The state of the art in 1987 is changing rapidly and is expected to improve greatly over the next few years. The authors give insight into the strengths and limitations of this new modality. They have liberally added examples of simultaneous 2D echocardiograms as well as pulsed and continuous-wave Doppler studies. This text/atlas is the first book completely dedicated to color flow imaging assessment of congenital heart disease and serves as an important introduction to this new and exciting technology.

James B. Seward, M.D.
Professor of Medicine,
Consultant, Cardiovascular Diseases
and Pediatric Cardiology,
Co-director, Echocardiography Laboratory,
Mayo Clinic, Rochester, Minnesota

Preface

Pediatric and adult cardiologists treating patients with congenital heart disease must obtain information concerning: (1) a detailed assessment of the *anatomy* of the congenital heart defect, and (2) an understanding of the *hemodynamics* and the abnormal physiology.

Echocardiography has had a major impact on understanding the anatomy of congenital heart disease and recent developments with pulsed and continuous-wave Doppler make a noninvasive hemodynamic assessment a reasonable possibility for the future. Color Doppler display of intracardiac and extracardiac blood flows gives a visual representation of the blood flow velocities of the heart. There are many who believe that color Doppler will be to pulsed Doppler echocardiography what two-dimensional echocardiography was to M-mode echo with regard to its impact on understanding abnormal physiology.

Color Doppler in Congenital Heart Disease will aid all who treat patients with congenital heart defects, including pediatric cardiologists, adult cardiologists, cardiac surgeons, intensive care physicians, and radiologists. Over 150 color illustrations elucidate the complex flow relationships in congenital heart defects and the pulsed Doppler and continuous-wave Doppler correlates are illustrated.

This text-atlas illustrates the most common hemodynamic abnormalities seen with congenital heart disease, in both the child and the adult, and the state of the art of color Doppler and its proven and likely impact. The principal emphasis is on communicating the abnormal physiology of the congenital cardiac abnormality, including stenotic valve lesions, regurgitant valves, left-to-right shunts, right-to-left shunts causing cyanosis with complex congenital heart disease, severe ventricular dysfunction (cardiomyopathy), and fetal echocardiography. Selected from an experience of over 2,000 color Doppler examinations in patients with congenital heart disease seen at the Echocardiography Laboratory at Texas Children's Hospital, the examples illustrate the strength of combining color Doppler with pulsed and continuous-wave Doppler techniques.

Because of the rapid explosion in technological developments in color Doppler, the illustrations include examples from three different manufacturers of color Doppler equipment. Technical limitations, and pitfalls in the day-to-day practical diagnosis of congenital heart disease with color flow mapping are discussed.

It is our hope that this project will expand the application of color Doppler flow mapping to congenital heart disease while maintaining a high-quality segmental anatomical approach to noninvasive diagnosis with echocardiography.

Achi Ludomirsky, M.D.
James C. Huhta, M.D.

Acknowledgments

This text-atlas could not have been completed without the diligent contributions of Grace Y. Yoon who organized the manuscript and helped in all aspects of the writing. We gratefully acknowledge the help of the Texas Children's Hospital Echocardiography Laboratory personnel, including Heidi Elder, Lucy C. Tabrizi, R.C.T., Dora V. Hewes, R.D.M.S., L.V.N., Regina Hanson, R.D.M.S., L.V.N., and Michelle Shotlow. We thank Drs. A. Khan and S. A. Yousef of the Armed Forces Hospital, Saudi Arabia, Michelle Dunn, G. Wesley Vick III, M.D., Ph.D., and the fellows and staff of the Section of Pediatric Cardiology, Baylor College of Medicine and Texas Children's Hospital.

We acknowledge the manufacturers who contributed in a significant way to the production of this text including Advanced Technology Laboratories, Corometrics-Aloka, Diasonics, Inc., Toshiba America, Inc., and Hewlett-Packard, Inc.

Our thanks to Steven Korn, Jacques Strauss, and Bessie Blum of Futura Publishing Company.

Without the support of two special people this project would not have been completed: Dan G. McNamara, M.D., Chief of Pediatric Cardiology, and Ralph D. Feigin, M.D., Chairman of Pediatrics, Baylor College of Medicine.

Grant Support

This work was supported in part by Grant RR-00188 from the General Clinical Research Branch, National Institutes of Health, Bethesda, Maryland, and by Grant RR-05425 from the National Institutes of Health, United States Public Health Service, Bethesda, Maryland, and by New Investigator Research Award HL31153 from the National Heart, Lung, and Blood Institute, United States Public Health Service.

To our wives and parents

Contents

Chapter 1

Basic Principles and Technical Considerations

David A. Danford, M.D.

The cardiac diagnostic process in congenital heart disease must involve the identification of anatomical abnormalities and the characterization of their pathophysiological consequences. Whatever diagnostic modalities the cardiologist chooses, these two aspects, anatomy and physiology, must be addressed as completely and as accurately as possible. In much the same way as cardiac angiography (anatomy) and catheterization (physiology) fit together in cardiologic diagnosis, two-dimensional and Doppler echocardiography are diagnostically complementary techniques. For well over a decade, two-dimensional echocardiographic imaging has provided the details of cardiac anatomy in congenital heart disease. Pulsed and continuous-wave Doppler echocardiography have added physiological details unavailable with imaging alone. Synthesis of the two aspects of echocardiographic diagnosis into a single real-time display by showing the Doppler information as a color overlay has theoretical appeal which has prompted considerable efforts to develop the technology to achieve it. These efforts have produced a method known by many names, including color Doppler echocardiography. The term "color flow mapping" is a misnomer because most color displays show blood cell velocity and not volume flow. We prefer the term "color Doppler" because it refers to the general technique of integrating hemodynamic information into the ultrasonic image using color. The remainder of this chapter is devoted to a review of the technology involved in producing color Doppler, and a discussion of the strengths and weaknesses of the technology in achieving a synthesis of the anatomical and physiological data required by the cardiologist.

The Doppler Principle

Color Doppler, like all of Doppler echocardiography, is based on a principle described by Christian Johann Doppler in 1842. He reported that the observed frequency of reflected waves coming from an object will increase if the object and observer are moving toward one another, and decrease if they are moving away (Figure 1-1). Although this principle applies generally to waves of all kinds and is true whether object, observer, or both are moving, it applies to echocardiography in the specific case of ultrasound reflected from objects moving with respect to a stationary receiver. Ultrasound reflected from moving blood cells returns to the observer at a higher frequency when the cells are moving toward the observer and at a lower frequency when they move away from the observer (Figure 1-2). The faster the blood cells move toward or away from the observer, the greater the effect on the observed frequency of the reflected ultrasound. Doppler echocardiography, then, is the diagnostic technique that draws inferences about blood velocity and direction of flow on the basis of differences between the transmitted and reflected frequency of ultrasound.[1] Accurate translation of a frequency shift of reflected ultrasound into a velocity requires (1) an assumption that the object is moving relative to the observer, (2) a knowledge of the velocity of sound transmission in what is presumed to be a homogeneous medium, and (3) information about the depth of the object.

Doppler echocardiography may be based either on the reflection of continuously transmitted ultrasound (continuous-wave Doppler) or on the reflection of intermittently transmitted ultrasound (pulsed Doppler) (Figure 1-3). Color Doppler is a specific form of presentation of pulsed Doppler data, and therefore is subject not only to the constraints and technical considerations that accompany Doppler echocardiography in general, but also to the peculiarities of pulsed Doppler. Some of the considerations that are of particular importance to the interpretation of color Doppler include: (1) angle of incidence of the ultrasound beam on the direction of

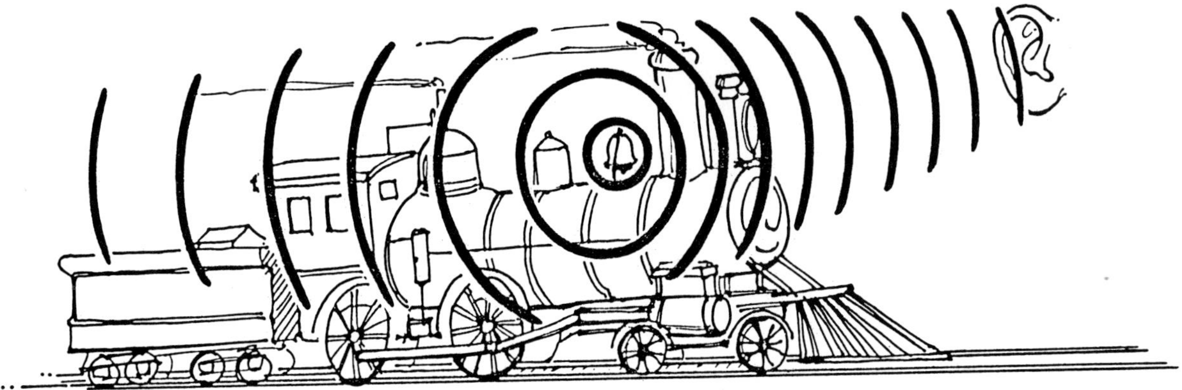

FIGURE 1-1—*The Doppler principle. Sound waves originating from a source (train whistle) moving toward the observer (ear) reach the ear at a higher frequency (waves closer together) than they would have had the source been stationary relative to the ear. Conversely, sound waves originating from a source moving away from the observer reach the ear at a lower frequency than they would have from a stationary source.*

blood flow; (2) velocity ambiguity versus range ambiguity; and (3) frequency dispersion within a sample.

Pulsed Doppler Echocardiography

Pulsed Doppler echocardiography transmits ultrasound in pulses at a known frequency. Between pulses, reflected ultrasound is received and the frequency of the reflected ultrasound is compared with the frequency transmitted. The difference between transmitted and received frequency (the frequency shift) indicates the direction and velocity of the blood cells. The faster the blood cells move toward or away from the observer, the greater the frequency shift.

Angle of Incidence

The Doppler principle applies only to motion toward or away from the observer. Movement of an object, no matter how rapid, in a direction that maintains a constant distance between object and observer produces no frequency shift (Figure 1-2c). This is true because the frequency shift produced by motion of blood cells is proportional not only to the velocity with which they are moving, but also to the cosine of the angle of incidence of the ultrasound with the vector of motion. A zero angle of incidence (ultrasound beam parallel to blood flow) has a cosine of one, whereas a 90-degree angle of incidence has a cosine of zero. It is important to remember that angle of incidence has an effect not only in the two dimensions displayed on the echocardiographic image but also to the third dimension out of the plane of imaging. This factor applies to color Doppler as well as conventional pulsed and continuous-wave Doppler echocardiography, and all have implications for the application of frequency shift of reflected ultrasound to determine the velocity of blood flow. We shall see that the color Doppler display format in fact does not correct for angle, and this must be taken into account by the echocardiographer interpreting the color Doppler display.

Velocity or Range Ambiguity

Pulsed Doppler echocardiography is a range-gated technique. In other words, frequency shifts are analyzed at a particular sample depth based on the anticipated transit time of ultrasound to the sample depth and back (Figure 1-3). Thus, pulsed Doppler detects frequency shifts of reflected ultrasound at a specific point of interest within the cardiovascular system which the echocardiographer can select. Pulsed Doppler, however, has built-in limitations in the specificity with which it can detect frequency shifts and the range at which they occur. Detection of the unique frequency shift depends on the sampling rate of the system. The faster the sampling rate, the larger the frequency shift that can be identified. In pulsed Doppler, sampling takes place only between pulses, so sampling is only as rapid as the pulse repetition frequency. The pulse repetition frequency, therefore, determines the frequency shifts which pulsed Doppler echocardiography can measure. Any frequency shift that exceeds one-half of the pulse repetition frequency cannot be identified uniquely (Figure 1-4a). In practical terms, this means that some physiological and many pathological blood flow velocities cannot be estimated using conventional pulsed Doppler echocardiography because the frequency shifts they produce are too large. Most pulsed Doppler echocardiographic systems display

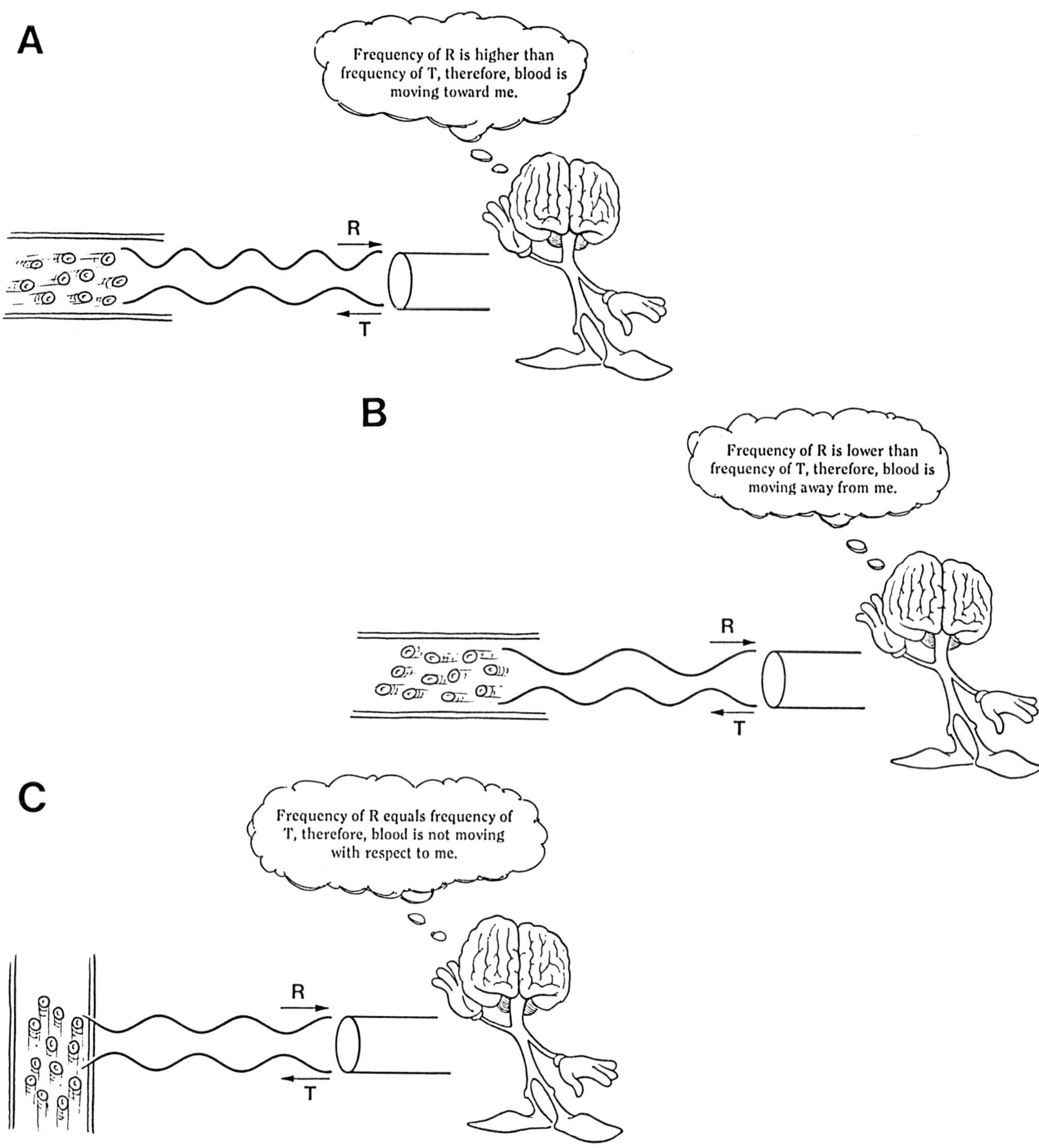

FIGURE 1-2—*(a) Blood cells moving toward the echocardiography transducer meet the transmitted ultrasound T. The ultrasound reflected by the cells R reaches the transducer at a higher frequency than T. The echocardiograph interprets the difference in frequencies R > T to mean the blood is moving toward the transducer. (b) Blood cells moving away from the transducer produce a reflected ultrasound wave R with a lower frequency than the transmitted wave T. The echocardiograph interprets the difference in frequencies R < T to mean the blood is moving away from the transducer. (c) Blood cells moving perpendicular to transmitted ultrasound wave T reflect it to the transducer with a frequency identical to T. The echocardiograph interprets the equality R = T to mean the blood is moving neither toward nor away from the transducer.*

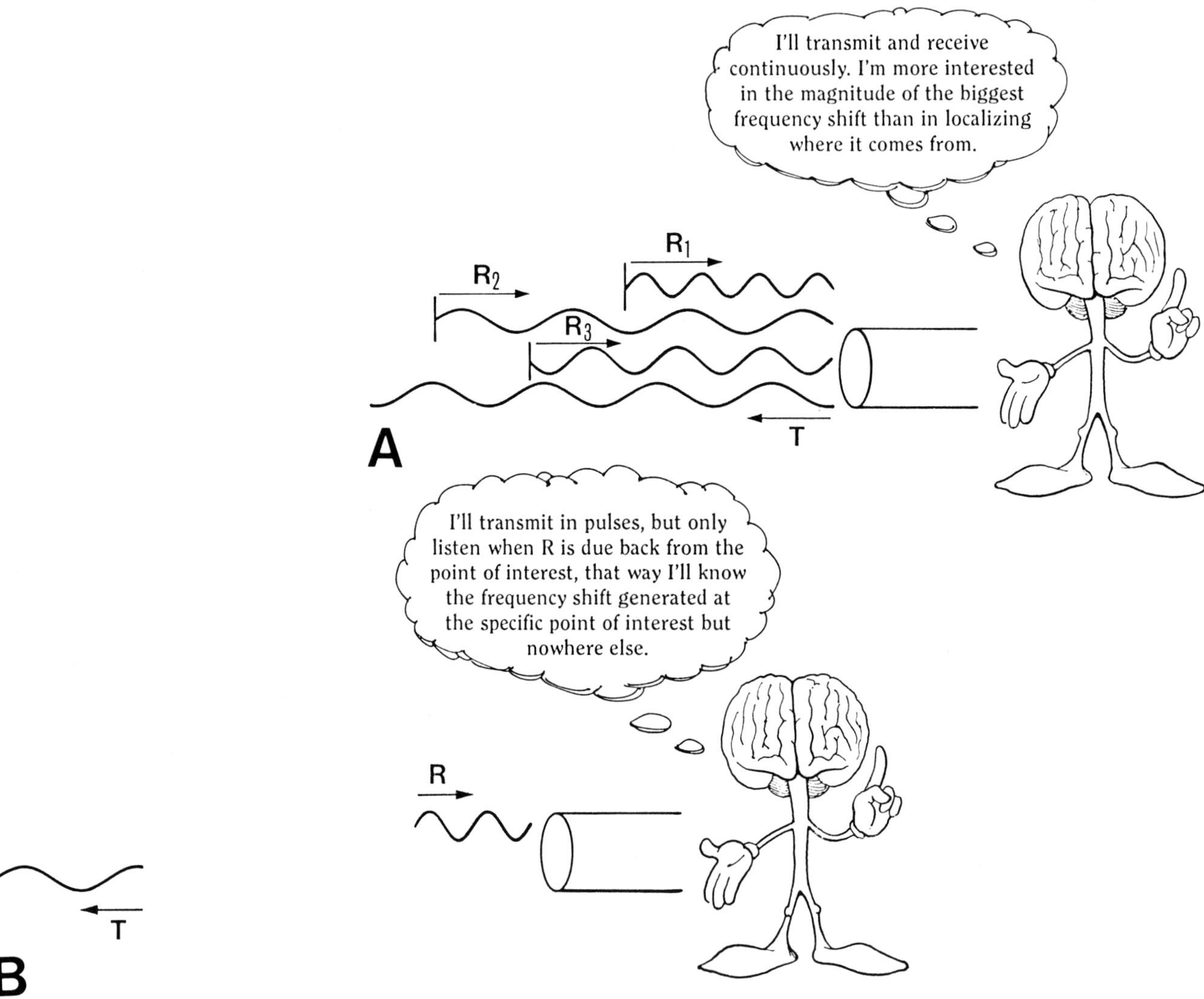

FIGURE 1-3—*Continuous-wave and pulsed Doppler. (a) Continuous-wave Doppler transmits and receives continuously. Reflected waves of many different frequencies (R1, R2, R3, . . .) originate from many locations along the transmitted wave. (b) Pulsed Doppler transmits and receives intermittently. The location from which the reflected wave originates can be established by knowing the speed of sound and the time elapsed since transmission of the pulse (range gating).*

these large frequency shifts by a convention known as aliasing, in which they are superimposed on the display of smaller frequency shifts.

Increasing the pulse repetition frequency would appear to be a potential solution to the problem of velocity ambiguity. Higher pulse repetition frequency, however, merely exchanges velocity ambiguity for range ambiguity. Because of the high pulse repetition frequency, more than one pulse of ultrasound will be in the heart at a given time. It will therefore be uncertain from which pulse at which location the returning ultrasound is reflected (Figure 1-4b). Range ambiguity, as we will see, is more confusing than velocity ambiguity in the color Doppler format, so color Doppler systems tend to have low pulse repetition frequencies. Furthermore, the greater the distance at which one samples, the lower the pulse repetition frequency must be to avoid range ambiguity. This is simply because of the longer ultrasound transit time to and from the deeper sampling site that must elapse before another pulse can be transmitted. The consequence of this is that the maximum uniquely identifiable blood velocities are lower when the sampling site is more distant.

Frequency Dispersion

In pulsed Doppler echocardiography, the size of the sampling site is large (usually several millimeters) com-

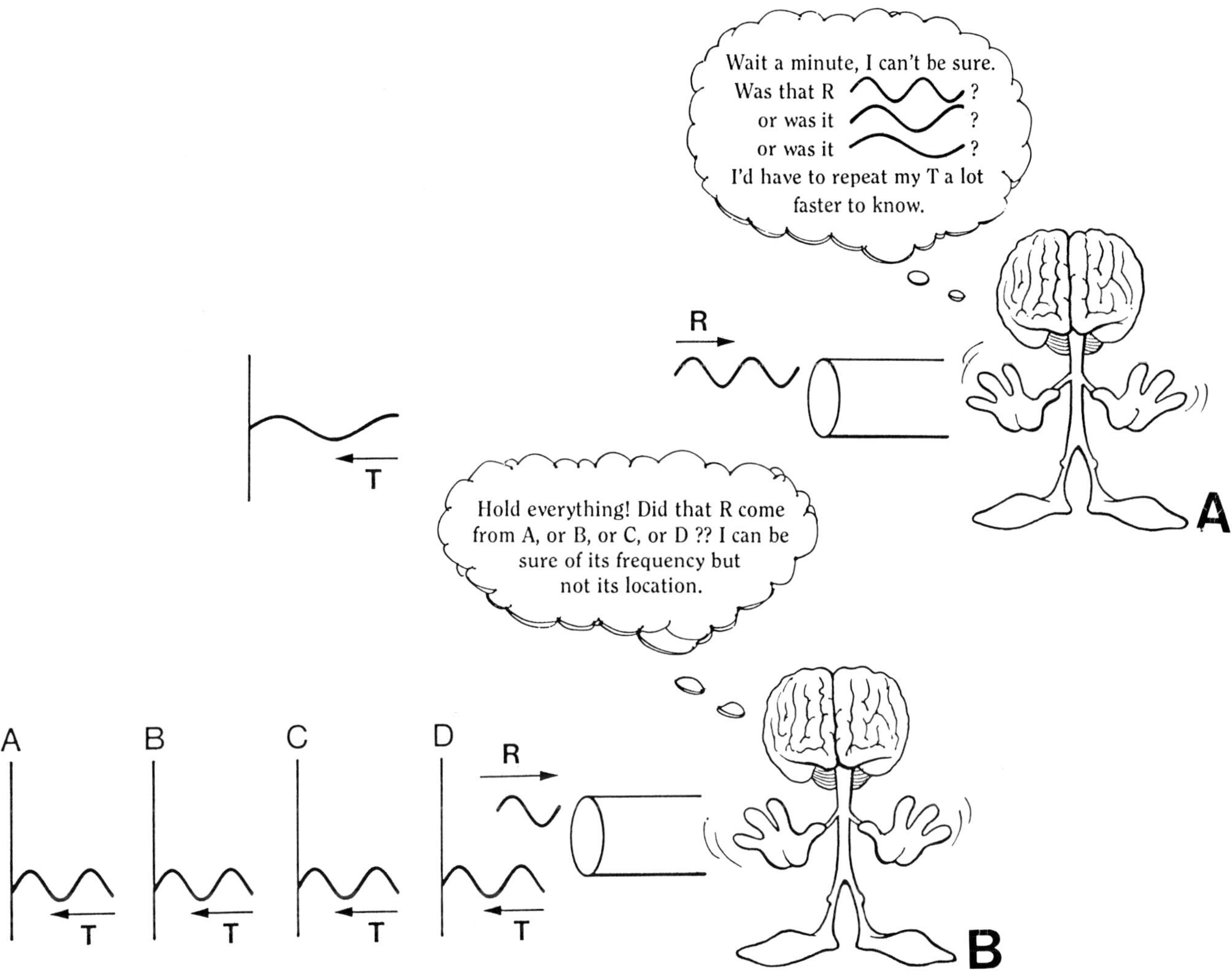

FIGURE 1-4—*Frequency and range ambiguity. (a) Pulsed Doppler is limited in its capacity to establish unequivocally the frequency of reflected ultrasound by the rate at which it can sample it. Large frequency shifts cannot be identified with certainty using conventional pulsed Doppler (frequency or velocity ambiguity). (b) The sampling rate of pulsed Doppler may be enhanced dramatically by increasing the rate at which it transmits pulses. This, however, results in the presence of multiple pulses of transmitted ultrasound in the heart at any given time and the point of origin of reflected ultrasound cannot be determined uniquely (range ambiguity).*

pared with the size of the moving objects (blood cells) from which the ultrasound is reflected. Because of the sample to target size disparity, very many moving blood cells are contained within the sample, each producing its own frequency shift. With laminar blood flow, most of the cells are moving at approximately the same speed and in approximately the same direction so the frequency shift signal produced is relatively pure. However, when flow is turbulent, blood cells are moving at different velocities and in different directions, reflecting ultrasound with many different frequency shifts (Figure 1-5). The greater the turbulence of blood flow, the greater the variability of frequency shifts (*frequency dispersion*) detected by pulsed Doppler. We shall see how frequency dispersion is incorporated into color Doppler display presentation.

Color Doppler Echocardiography

Color Doppler is a display format that combines two-dimensional echocardiographic imaging with pulsed Doppler data from many points within the image. The Doppler information is coded by color and brightness and presented to the echocardiographer simultaneously with the anatomical information.[2-8] The display in

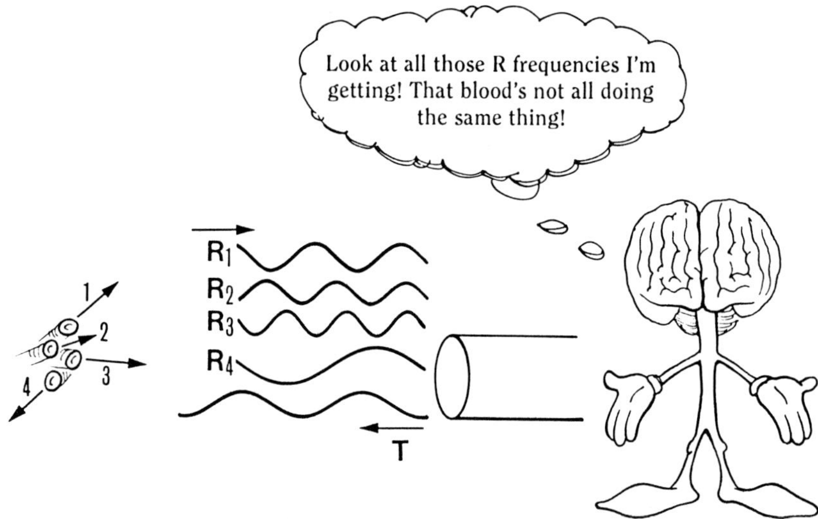

FIGURE 1-5—*Frequency dispersion. The "range" in range-gated pulsed Doppler is not a precise point but has length, width, and depth. It therefore contains many moving blood cells. When there is considerable variability among these cells with respect to direction and velocity, there are a variety of different reflected frequencies (R1, R2, R3, . . .).*

most common use today combines the two-dimensional echocardiogram with color coding of Doppler velocities. We will discuss this format first, but it is by no means the only potential presentation format for color Doppler. The display of Doppler data superimposed on the M-mode echocardiogram, or the mapping of Doppler power density function instead of velocity on the two-dimensional echocardiogram are technologically feasible alternative presentations of color Doppler. These will be discussed later.

The major obstacle to be overcome in the production of a real-time display of Doppler data from many sampling sites along many scan lines is the long time required for signal processing of Doppler by conventional fast Fourier transform (FFT) methods.[9-11] Processing Doppler data from each individual radial scan line using an FFT takes a minimum of 20 milliseconds per scan line to achieve satisfactory frequency resolution. The number of scan lines that could be generated using an FFT during the time period between frames using even a very slow, choppy frame rate would be too small to produce a meaningful picture.

A different signal processing technique was first applied to produce the color Doppler display in less than one-tenth the time taken by the FFT. The reflected signal is passed first through a *quadrature* detector which converts the received waveform to one that is 90 degrees out of phase with the original. The unaltered received waveform and the 90 degrees out-of-phase waveform are multiplied by the transmitted wave form to allow calculation of the frequency shift of the received wave from the transmitted. Because of frequency dispersion, the frequency shift is variable within any sampling site along the scan line. To interpret this variable frequency shift, an *autocorrelator* consisting of a time delay circuit and multiplier is used to obtain a *mean* and a *variance* for the frequency shifts supplied by the quadrature detector. The output of the autocorrelator is integrated over a number of transmission cycles to increase the signal-to-noise ratio. The output of this signal-processing system is a mean and variance of the frequency shift at each of many individual points along each of many scan lines (Figure 1-6).

The direction of flow is coded by color, red for flow toward the observer, and blue for flow away from the observer. The velocity of flow is coded by brightness, with the brighter blue or red hues representing faster velocities. The Doppler output is superimposed on a two-dimensional image, producing a flow map which is presented to the echocardiographer. The flow map can be displayed on a television screen in real time or as an electrocardiographically time-gated image at a particular point in the cardiac cycle. Because of the rapidity with which the echocardiographer is bombarded with data in the real-time color Doppler display, the gated mode has proven very useful in congenital heart disease. The flow map may be recorded in either of these formats on video tape for storage and later review.

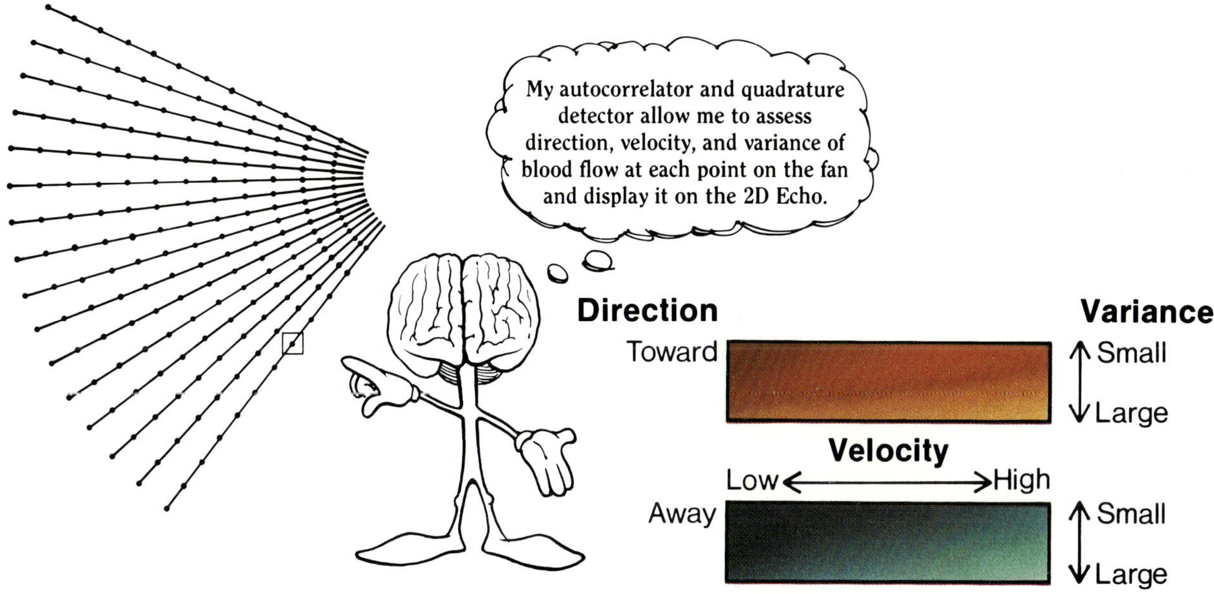

FIGURE 1-6—*Color Doppler echocardiography. New signal processing techniques allow determination of flow direction, velocity, and variance at many points simultaneously, rapidly enough to show them in real-time with the two-dimensional image. Conventional coding for direction is red or blue by color, velocity by brightness, and variance by injection of yellow or cyan.*

Technical Interpretative Considerations

The three major interpretative considerations of pulsed Doppler echocardiography discussed previously (angle of incidence, velocity/range ambiguity, and frequency dispersion) all have impact on the interpretation of the color Doppler display. The color Doppler display does not correct for the *angle of incidence* of the ultrasonic beam with the direction of blood flow. The echocardiographer must make allowances for the fact that a zero angle of incidence is assumed by the color Doppler machine for the velocities it displays. Therefore, the velocity of blood flow is often underestimated by relying on its presentation in the color Doppler format.

The presentation of color Doppler is a flow map in which a one-to-one correspondence between points on the map and displayed signals is maintained. *Range ambiguity*, in which a given signal would be displayed at more than one point, would produce an uninterpretable map. Therefore, *velocity ambiguity* (aliasing) is chosen as a lesser of two evils for use in the color-flow display. High-velocity aliasing signals approaching the observer are shown in blue, not the conventional red. Conversely, aliasing signals going away from the transducer are displayed as red, not the conventional blue. Because of its relatively slow pulse repetition rate, color Doppler is particularly prone to aliasing.

Finally, *frequency dispersion* is determined as the variance of the signal by the autocorrelator. It is added to the velocity signal as an alternate hue such as green, which makes the turbulent blood flow appear not as a pure red or blue, but as a distinctive speckled yellow or cyan.

Other technical considerations affect the design of color Doppler systems and the output that they present to the echocardiographer. Some systems, for example, allow the echocardiographer a choice of eliminating the variance coding (turbulence) at the touch of a switch, producing a somewhat different appearance (Figure 1-7). It is also possible, although not necessarily advisable, to reverse the red and blue coding on some color Doppler systems so that red indicates flow away and blue indicates flow toward the transducer. Early experience with color Doppler using mechanical sector scanners has been hindered by an artifact in which stationary objects are perceived as producing Doppler shifts because of the movement of the receiver relative to the object. Because of difficulty overcoming this, most color Doppler systems use phased array transducers.

Ultrasound exposure of the duration, frequency, intensity, and power used in clinical echocardiographic imaging and Doppler examination has never been shown to be hazardous to infants, children, or adults. Color Doppler does not produce significantly higher exposure, and so would not be expected to be hazardous. Special safety considerations are prudent for fetal Doppler examinations in general, and these carry over to color Doppler (see Chapter 11).

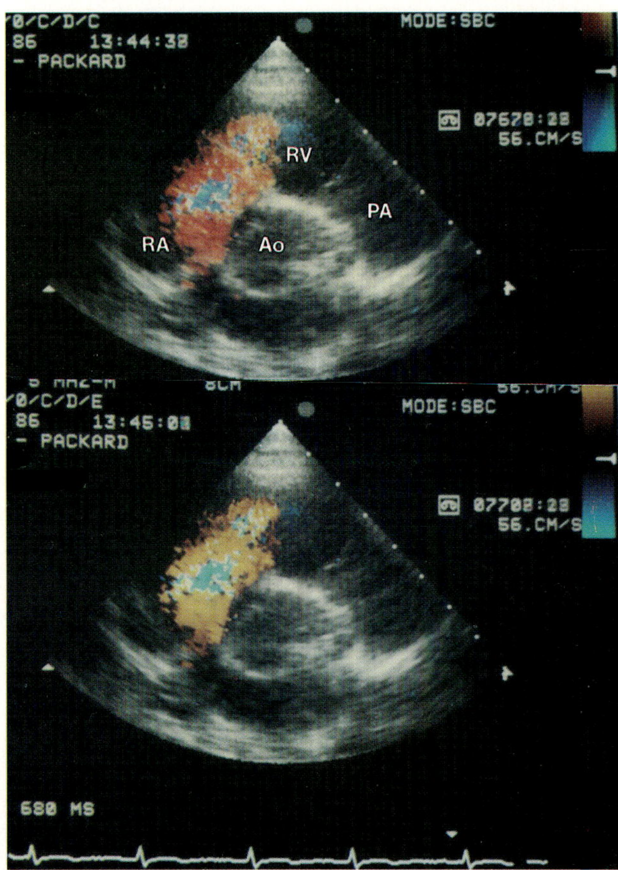

FIGURE 1-7—*Elimination of variance. Injection of yellow speckles into the red pattern of right ventricular inflow indicates variance in detected frequency shifts by color Doppler in the upper panel. The lower panel shows the same right ventricular inflow without variance display. Here, yellow is used to indicate higher velocity. Note that both formats show aliasing with a blue signal. Ao = aorta; PA = pulmonary artery; RA = right atrium; RV = right ventricle.*

Trade-offs

A complex trade-off relationship exists between the number of scan lines, the number of pulses averaged (Doppler signal-to-noise ratio), depth of imaging, and the frame rate of the display. Because of the time required for ultrasound transmission and signal processing, if any of these four factors is increased, one of the others must decrease or the flow map could not be completed in the time between frames. Technical design compromise is required to produce adequate scan-line density, frame rate, frequency resolution, and depth of scan, in which no feature is sacrificed excessively (Figure 1-8). In a practical sense, this can have a number of implications. For example, the resolution of the color flow map image is poorer than when two-dimensional imaging is used alone because of decreased frame rate or reduced density of scan lines. On the other hand, faster frame rate or greater density of scan lines may be produced by narrowing the width of the sector in which color flow mapping is done. It is also of practical concern that the color flow map image is degraded with color Doppler examination at great depth because a decreased frame rate, decreased number of scan lines, or a decreased number of pulses averaged is needed to compensate for the greater length of transit time required to scan at greater depths.

Blood Flow versus Wall Motion

It would be distracting for a color Doppler display to code heart wall and valve motion in color in addition to coding blood flow in color. A filter to eliminate low-velocity, high-amplitude Doppler signals is incorporated into the system to prevent this. This filter, if it is effective, also eliminates some potentially important low-velocity blood flow signals. If the filter is less than entirely effective, the faint superimposition of color on moving cardiac tissue produces an annoying artifact called "ghosting" (Figure 1-9). Various algorithms for making the decision whether a velocity is heart wall or blood flow can be incorporated into the display. In congenital heart disease, a major application of color is detection of ventricular septal defects and a velocity map that makes blood flow seem to occur in the substance of the septum can lead to the false-positive diagnosis of muscular defect (see Chapter 5).

Unconventional Color Doppler Presentations

Until now we have discussed color Doppler in a limited sense, in that the imaging format was two-dimensional echocardiography and the Doppler format was velocity coding. There are other color Doppler presentations that may be useful in certain situations. Most systems allow the superimposition of color-coded Doppler velocities on an M-mode echocardiogram. This allows the precise timing of changes in direction and turbulence of blood flow along a single scan line (Figure 1-10).

Color Doppler M-mode format gives far better temporal resolution of flow patterns than is possible with the frame rate limitations of the color Doppler two-dimensional display. Color M-mode is valuable as a temporal scout which serves to locate in time the flow pattern of interest. Once the event of interest is precisely temporally located, the two-dimensional color Doppler display may be gated at that time of interest during the

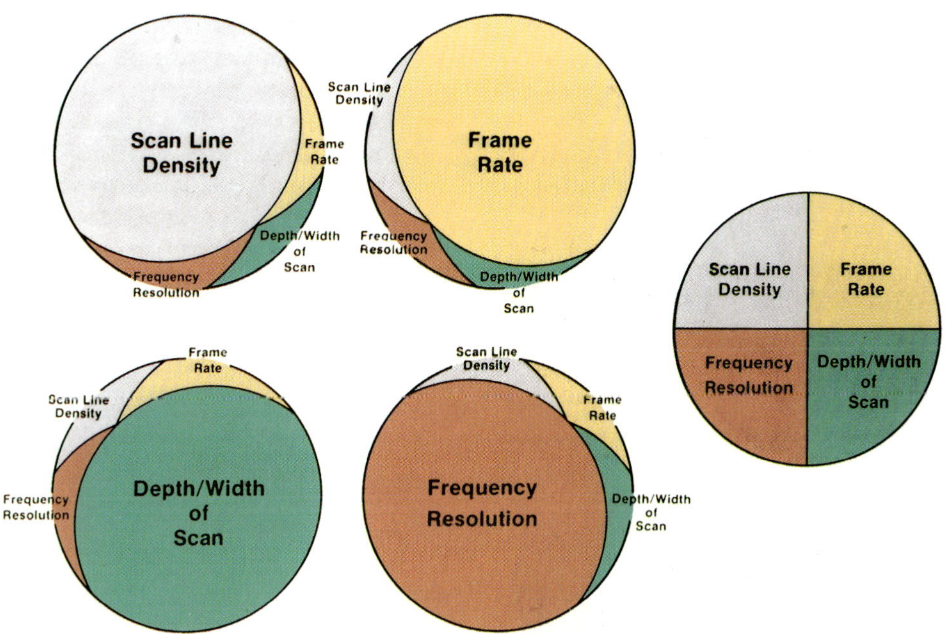

FIGURE 1-8—*Technical compromises. Color Doppler picture quality is dependent on four competing factors: scan-line density, frame rate, frequency resolution, and depth and width of the scan. It is not advisable to increase any one of these factors to the point that the others are sacrificed.*

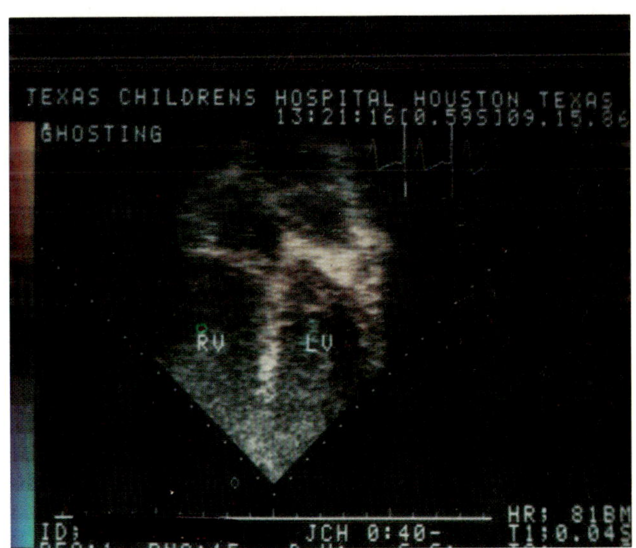

FIGURE 1-9—*Ghosting. The appearance of red color within the myocardium is an artifact called ghosting. LV = left ventricle; RV = right ventricle.*

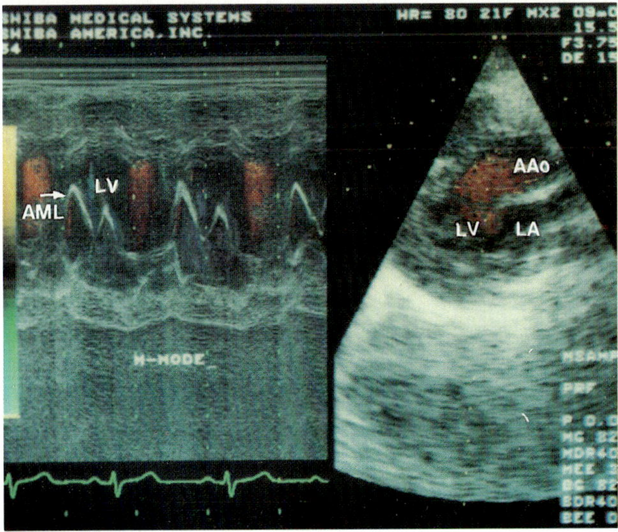

FIGURE 1-10—*Color M-mode. The color M-mode display can improve the temporal resolution of color Doppler. At left, a color M-mode of left ventricular inflow and outflow occurring on either side of the anterior mitral valve leaflet demonstrates this. As in more conventional formats, red indicates flow toward the transducer (in this case systolic left ventricular outflow) and blue indicates flow away from the transducer (here diastolic left ventricular inflow). A systolic frame from the parasternal long-axis two-dimensional color Doppler is shown at right for comparison. AAo = ascending aorta; AML = anterior mitral leaflet; LA = left atrium; LV = left ventricle.*

cardiac cycle, and the flow signal may be more completely mapped and characterized.

Another color Doppler format is power function (intensity) mapping. The direction of blood flow is coded using the standard red and blue system for flow toward and away from the observer. The intensity or power density function rather than the velocity of the Doppler flow signal is coded by the brightness of the display (Figure 1-11). Low-velocity, high-volume flow such as that in the atria, pulmonary veins, or systemic veins is better seen in this format than with velocity mapping. Similarly, the extent and volume of flows such as mitral or tricuspid regurgitation would be more accurately estimated this way, since they reflect a regurgitant volume rather than a regurgitant jet velocity (see Chapter 4). This mode is also less restrictive with regard to angle problems because of increased sensitivity to lower velocities. High-velocity flow is not coded by aliasing and is indistinguishable from low-velocity flow in this format. Because of its selection of low-velocity high-intensity signals, ghosting would be expected to be a particular problem with this presentation. In actual practice, ghosting in this format can usually be eliminated by reducing the gain, without eliminating the blood flow signals of interest.

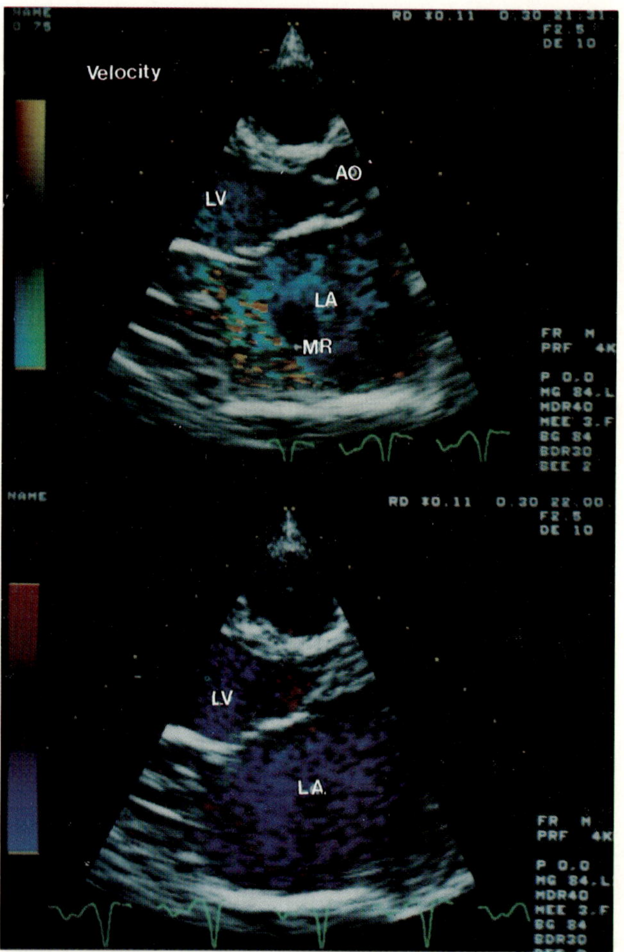

FIGURE 1-11—*Intensity function mapping. The color Doppler display above shows conventional velocity coded format. Below is the intensity function coded format. Note the differences in appearance due to absence of aliasing and variance in the intensity mode. The mitral regurgitation jet appears more extensive using intensity mode. Ao = aorta; LA = left atrium; LV = left ventricle; MR = mitral regurgitation.*

Technical Directions for the Future

Although the development of the color Doppler system as a useful diagnostic tool that combines anatomical and physiological information in a single display is in its infancy, it already seems likely that color Doppler will be to pulsed Doppler what two-dimensional was to M-mode echocardiography.[12-16] To fulfill this prophesy, many obstacles must be overcome. The quality of the two-dimensional anatomical display, in terms of its scan-line density and frame rate, needs substantial improvement. Furthermore, the optimal mode for display of Doppler data has not yet been developed. It is likely that the optimal display format will, with experience, be tailored for the particular physiological setting. Perhaps some imaginative combination of display of power density function and velocity will provide a physiological display that the clinician would find relevant. A problem that will continue to confound color Doppler is aliasing at low velocities, which prevents the display of clinically important peak flow velocities of high-velocity jets. Incorporation of continuous-wave Doppler data simultaneously into the color Doppler display format would increase the clinical power of the technique. Despite these limitations, color Doppler techniques are now being applied for the evaluation of congenital heart disease in an increasing number of centers throughout the world. It remains to be seen to what extent color Doppler will fulfill its promise as the "compleat" noninvasive anatomical and physiological diagnostic tool, and if it will, what new technology will be required to bring this about.

References

1. Hatle L, Angelsen B: Doppler Ultrasound in Cardiology—Physical Principles and Clinical Applications, 2nd ed. Philadelphia, Lea & Febiger, 1985.
2. Switzer DF, Nanda NC: Doppler color flow mapping. Ultrasound Med Biol 3:403-416, 1985.
3. Sahn DJ: Real-time 2-dimensional Doppler echocardiographic flow mapping. Circulation 71:849-853, 1985.
4. Schoenfeld, MR: Focus on: Color-coded, real-time, two-dimensional Doppler echocardiographic mapping of in-

tracardiac blood flow. J Cardiovasc Ultrasonography 4:3-4, 1985.
5. Nishimura RA, Miller FA Jr, Callahan MJ, et al: Doppler echocardiography: Theory, instrumentation, technique and application. Mayo Clin Proc 60:321-343, 1985.
6. Nimura Y, Miyatake K: Recent progress in ultrasonic diagnosis of the heart: Doppler flow imaging. Jpn Circ J 49:694-701, 1985.
7. Durell M, Nanda NC: Doppler color flow mapping. In Nanda NC (ed): Doppler Echocardiography. New York, Igaku-Shoin Medical, 1985, p 515-516.
8. Iimuma K, Seo Y, Skirasaka T, et al: Real-time two-dimensional ultrasound blood flow imaging system. J Ultrasound Med 2:6, 1983 (abstr).
9. Omoto R: Color Atlas of Real-Time Two Dimensional Doppler Echocardiography. Tokyo, Sinden-To-Chiryosha, 1983.
10. Namekawa K, Kasai C, Tsukamoto M, Koyano A: Imaging of blood flow using auto-correlation. Ultrasound Med Biol 8:138, 1982 (abstr).
11. Bommer WJ: Basic principles of flow imaging. Echocardiography 2:501-509, 1985.
12. Roelandt J: Colour-coded Doppler flow imaging: What are the prospects? Eur Heart J 7:184-189, 1986.
13. DeMaria AN, Smith MD, Kwan OK: Doppler flow imaging: Another step in the evolution of cardiac ultrasound. Echocardiography 2:495-500, 1985.
14. Goldman, ME: Real-time two-dimensional Doppler flow imaging: A word of caution. J Am Coll Cardiol 7:89-90, 1986.
15. Namekawa K, Kasai C, Tsukamoto M, Koyano A: Real-time two- dimensional blood flow imaging using ultrasound Doppler. J Ultrasound Med 2 (Suppl): 6, 1983.
16. Nishimura RA, Tajik AJ, Reeder GS, Seward JB: Evaluation of hypertrophic cardiomyopathy by Doppler color flow imaging: Initial observations. Mayo Clin Proc 61:631-639, 1986.

Chapter 2

The Normal Examination

David A. Danford, M.D.

Segmental Approach to Color Doppler in the Normal

With any diagnostic tool, recognition of the normal is an essential foundation for the detection of the abnormal. In two-dimensional echocardiography, for example, the examiner must recognize normal cardiovascular anatomy in order to identify abnormalities when they appear. The heart and great vessels form a complex structure, within which each component may be normal or abnormal. Therefore, complete examination of each component of the heart and great vessels and recognition of its normality is required before the entire echocardiogram can be declared to be normal. Pathologists, angiocardiographers, and echocardiographers have found such "segmental analysis" of the heart to be a useful approach to this complicated problem. Integration of color flow data into the two- dimensional echocardiogram adds physiological information, which in combination with the anatomy, must be recognized as normal or abnormal in each segment of the heart.

Beginning at the systemic venous level and proceeding along the normal path of blood flow, this chapter introduces the normal color flow echocardiogram one segment at a time. Synthesis of these normal color flow segments provides a concept of the complete color Doppler echocardiogram in the normal.[1-5] Against this constructed image of normal, the abnormalities described in the remainder of this book stand in contrast.

Blood flow in the superior vena cava is high volume and moderate velocity. It proceeds toward the heart at velocities that vary with the phase of the cardiac cycle without sustained periods of flow reversal. A very brief period of flow reversal in the superior vena cava may follow atrial systole. Accordingly, the color Doppler echocardiogram obtained from the suprasternal notch transducer position demonstrates a blue signal throughout the superior vena cava and proximal innominate vein (Figure 2-1). Evidence of mild turbulent flow (injection of green into the homogeneous blue signal) may be seen. High-velocity flow producing aliasing (the appearance of red signal within the blue) is unusual. Because some color Doppler systems are relatively insensitive to low-velocity flow, the detection of the blood flow signal in the superior vena cava may be quite dependent on the angle of interrogation. Furthermore, the signal may appear and disappear with the normal changes in velocity that occur throughout the cardiac cycle or the respiratory cycle. At no time, however, should sustained flow reversal be evident in the normal. Nor should a constant velocity be present instead of the usual phasic variation of flow velocity in the superior vena cava in the normal. Mapping of normal superior vena cava flow may require careful attention to gain and filter settings in order to produce a satisfactory flow map. This problem can be circumvented by using an intensity function color Doppler system (Chapter 1) to display this low-velocity flow.

With the transducer in the subcostal position, imaging the right and left atria and the atrial septum, flow in the superior vena cava as it enters the right atrium can be demonstrated. Superior vena cava flow comes toward the transducer in this position, and so is coded as red on the color Doppler echocardiogram (Figure 2-2). This flow signal in the normal is without evidence of high-velocity aliasing. With color Doppler, it is important to try to resolve the normal flow pattern of superior vena caval blood entering the right atrium from the abnormal flow pattern of blood entering the right atrium as distinct across an atrial septal defect (see Chapter 5). Inferior vena caval blood flow can be detected in this subcostal view of the atria as low-velocity blood flow away from the transducer can be detected within the right atrium directed toward (but not passing through) the fossa ovalis. In the atrial level short-axis cut obtained from the subcostal transducer position (Figure 2-2), this appears as a blue signal along the right side of the atrial septum. When the ultrasound beam is directed posteriorly from the subcostal position to produce a saggital image of the upper abdomen along the long axis of the inferior vena cava (Figure 2-3), inferior vena cava

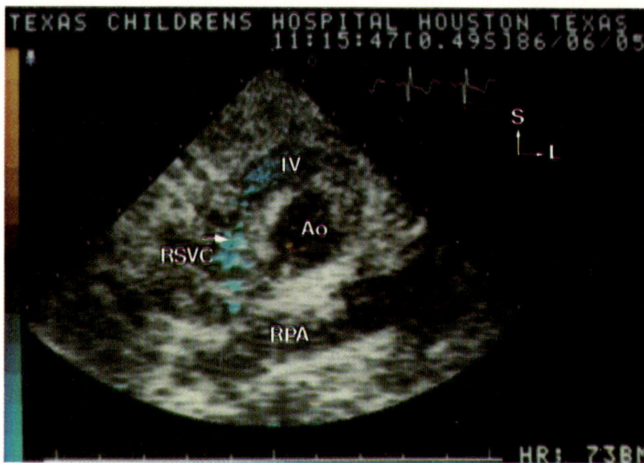

FIGURE 2-1—*Systemic venous return from the superior vena cava and innominate vein is detected travelling away from the transducer in the suprasternal notch position. This signal is coded in blue (flow away from transducer) without aliasing and with a moderate amount of frequency dispersion. Ao = aorta; L = left; IV = innominate vein; RPA = right pulmonary artery; RSVC = right superior vena cava; S = superior.*

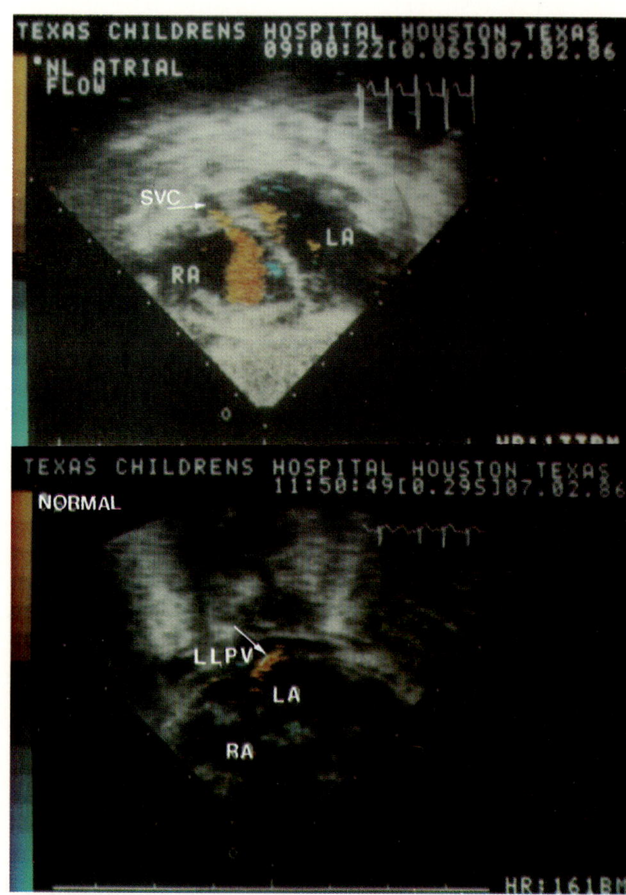

FIGURE 2-2—*In this subcostal short-axis view at the level of the atria (upper panel), superior vena caval flow occurs toward the transducer as it proceeds inferiorly into the right atrium. Occasionally a blue signal may be seen representing inferior vena caval flow directed superiorly and toward the atrial septum in this view. Pulmonary venous blood entering the left atrium is shown as a red signal flowing from the right upper pulmonary vein into the left atrium along the atrial septum. Note that no blood flow signals appear to cross the atrial septum in this normal example. Slight angulation of the transducer from the standard atrial level short-axis view may bring into view signals of flow entering the left atrium from other pulmonary veins. The lower panel shows a red signal originating from blood flow in the left lower pulmonary vein directed toward the transducer. LA = left atrium; LLPV = left lower pulmonary vein; RA = right atrium; SVC = superior vena cava.*

blood flows away from the transducer. This produces a homogeneous blue signal without frequency dispersion from turbulence, aliasing from high velocities, or time-dependent flow reversal in the normal. Hepatic venous flow is also directed away from the transducer in this position. This results in a homogeneous blue signal in the hepatic veins. Sustained flow reversal, particularly during ventricular systole, in the hepatic veins and inferior vena cava is not seen in the normal (see Chapter 10). Because inferior vena cava blood flow is low velocity and can be directed almost perpendicular to the direction of the ultrasound beam, it may be more difficult to map inferior vena cava blood flow than it is to map superior vena cava blood flow. Again, sensitive velocity mappers with high gain settings and low filter settings can produce adequate inferior vena cava flow maps. Intensity function mapping can be useful in this setting as well.

Right atrial[6] color Doppler in the normal is characterized by the normal inflow of blood from the inferior and superior vena cavae just described. Blood flow entering the right atrium across the atrial septum, through the coronary sinus ostium, or regurgitating back across the tricuspid insufficiency is potentially detectable in some normal individuals using sensitive color Doppler equipment, but is not usually prominent.[7] In addition to the signals from blood entering the right atrium normally from the inferior and superior vena cavae, right atrial color Doppler is characterized by the diastolic egress of blood from the right atrium across the tricuspid valve into the right ventricle. This tends to be somewhat faster blood flow than systemic venous flow; however, it is generally not fast enough to produce aliasing within the right atrium before it reaches the right ventricle. This diastolic flow of blood out of the right atrium can be demonstrated in several echocardiographic views, including the parasternal short-axis (Figure 2-4) and the apical four-chamber view. In these views diastolic flow leaving the right atrium across the tricuspid valve is seen as a red signal indicating blood flow toward the transducer.

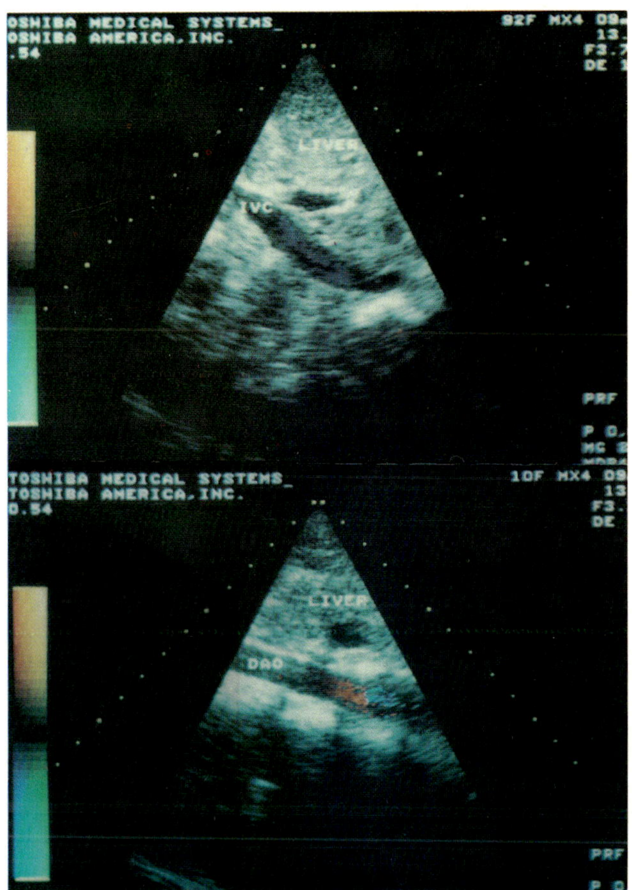

FIGURE 2-3—*With the transducer in the subcostal position, the scan plane is oriented along the long axis of the abdomen just to the right of midline (upper panel). Flow in the inferior vena cava is seen as a blue signal as it proceeds away from the transducer toward the heart. No aliasing and no frequency dispersion are seen. The plane of ultrasonic imaging is changed to the long axis of the abdominal aorta with the transducer in the subcostal position (lower panel). An inconsistent flow map is usual here, with some areas red, some blue, and some devoid of signal—largely depending on the direction of blood flow relative to the path of the ultrasound. DAo = descending aorta; IVC = inferior vena cava.*

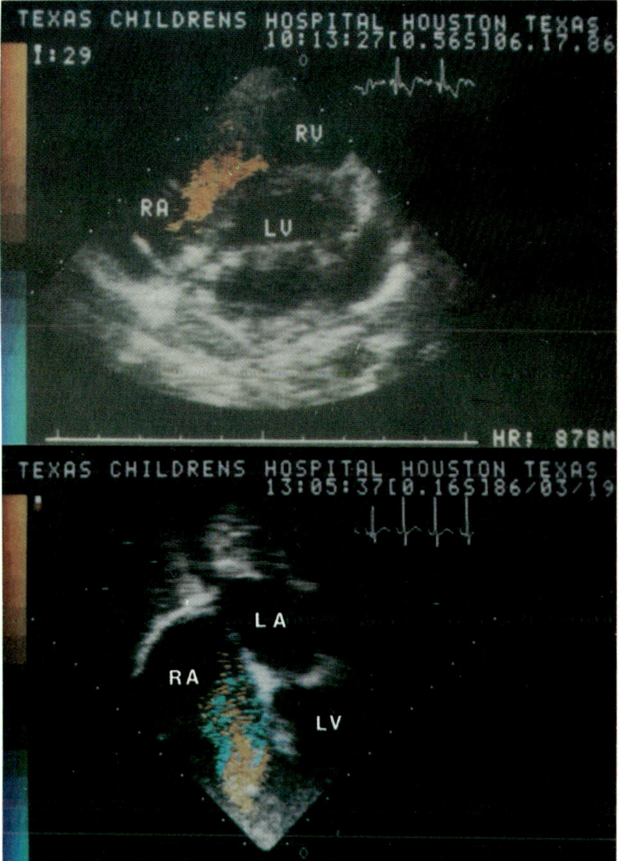

FIGURE 2-4—*Normal right ventricular (RV) inflow. Upper panel: in the parasternal transducer position with the scan plane oriented across the short axis of the heart at the level of the atrioventricular valves, diastolic right ventricular inflow can be seen. Right ventricular inflow is directed toward the transducer, producing a display coded red. Some frequency dispersion is present in this example, but there is no aliasing. Aliasing of this signal is relatively common in the normal. Lower panel: with the transducer near the cardiac apex, right ventricular diastolic inflow appears as a red signal with some frequency dispersion and aliasing. LV = left ventricle; RA = right atrium.*

The normal right ventricular color Doppler examination consists of two components: right ventricular inflow across the tricuspid valve and right ventricular outflow across the pulmonary valve. Right ventricular inflow can be mapped in diastole from any of several transducer positions, including the apical, parasternal, and subcostal. Right ventricular inflow is seen as a prominent red signal indicating blood flow toward the transducer in all of these locations. During early diastole (rapid filling), the velocity of blood entering the right ventricle may be fast enough to produce aliasing, particularly if mapping is done at a substantial depth from the transducer. Thus, as shown in Figure 2-4, there may be some blue signal centrally within an otherwise red inflow pattern. During slow filling, the aliasing pattern disappears because blood flow is at a quite low velocity during that time. Aliasing may reappear during the atrial kick at the end of diastole. Diastolic inflow across the tricuspid valve is the only source of blood entering the right ventricle detectable by color Doppler in the normal. Signals arising from the blood entering the right ventricle during diastole at a site other than the tricuspid valve (as in coronary fistula; see Chapter 9) or during systole across the ventricular septum (as in ventricular septal defect with left-to-right shunting [see Chapter 5] are abnormal).

During systole, the color Doppler detects blood flow in the right ventricular outflow tract travelling away from the transducer when the transducer is in the left parasternal (Figure 2-5) or subcostal position. In the normal, this flow shows some injection of green for frequency dispersion in the right ventricular outflow tract. This flow also can reach high velocity, so aliasing is common. In the normal, no jet of blood crosses the ventricular septum to enter the right ventricular outflow tract during systole (Figures 2-5 and 2-6).

The pulmonary valve, main pulmonary artery, and proximal left pulmonary artery may be imaged from the left infraclavicular or high left parasternal transducer position (Figure 2-6). In systole, a flow pattern is recorded in the main and left pulmonary arteries going away from the transducer. This signal will often alias because of the high velocity of blood flow, and there is usually some frequency dispersion. The presence of marked frequency dispersion in the main or left pulmonary artery should raise the question of a hemodynamic abnormality such as pulmonary stenosis or patent ductus arteriosus (see Chapters 3 and 10). Figure 2-6 shows the normal aliased but nonturbulent signal originating from the flow in the right and left pulmonary arteries. Normally, little or no flow signal arises from these structures in diastole; the presence of such a signal should suggest a naturally occurring or surgically created systemic to pulmonary artery shunt (see Chapters 8 and 10). With the transducer in the suprasternal notch, the proximal right pulmonary artery can be imaged somewhat better (Figure 2-7). In the

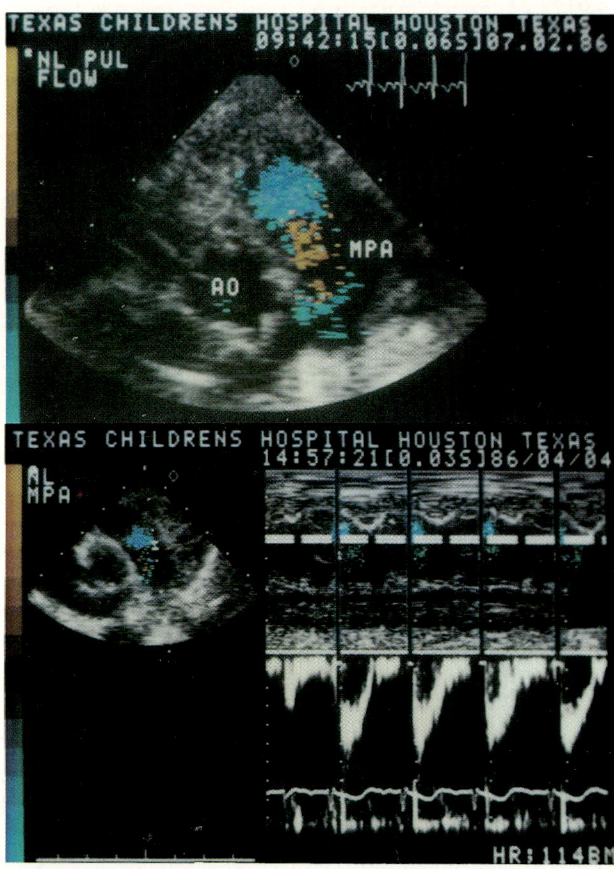

FIGURE 2-5—*Normal right ventricular outflow tract. With the transducer in the parasternal position and the plane of ultrasound directed toward the roots of the great arteries across the short axis of the heart, systolic flow is detected travelling away from the transducer in the right ventricular outflow tract and main pulmonary artery (upper panel). This flow is coded in blue with a substantial amount of central red aliasing. The lower panel shows corresponding pulsed Doppler recordings from the proximal main pulmonary artery. The location of the sample volume on the two- dimensional image is shown at left. The depth of the sample volume is also indicated by the interrupted line across the color M-mode display at right. AO = aorta; MPA = main pulmonary artery.*

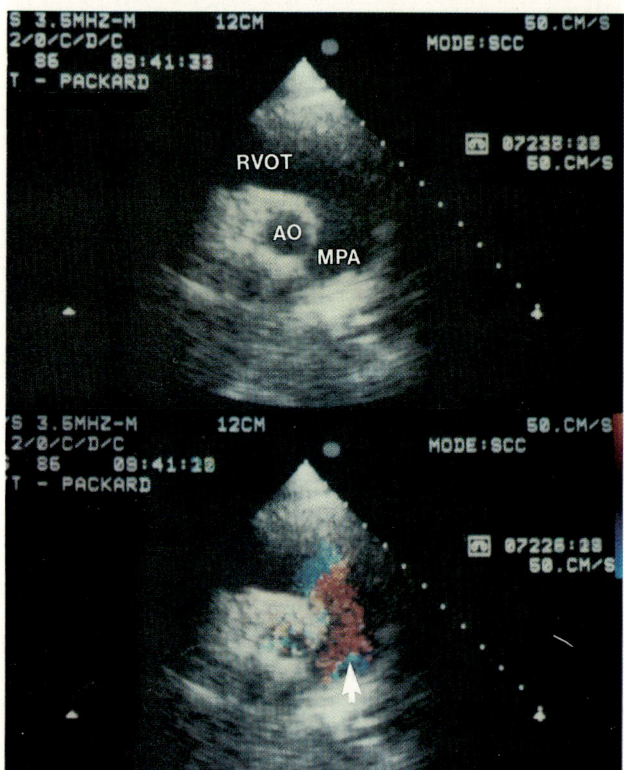

FIGURE 2-6—*Normal pulmonary arteries. This high left parasternal transducer position yields an image of the main pulmonary artery (MPA) and its bifurcation into the proximal right and left pulmonary arteries (white arrow in lower panel). The systolic flow in the main pulmonary artery is fast enough to alias quite prominently. This phenomenon is apparent also beyond the bifurcation of the pulmonary artery. Note there is no signal from blood crossing the interventricular septum to enter the right ventricular outflow tract in this normal example. The high velocities in the ascending aorta directed nearly perpendicular to the ultrasound produce marked frequency dispersion (mosaic pattern). AO = aorta; RVOT = right ventricular outflow tract.*

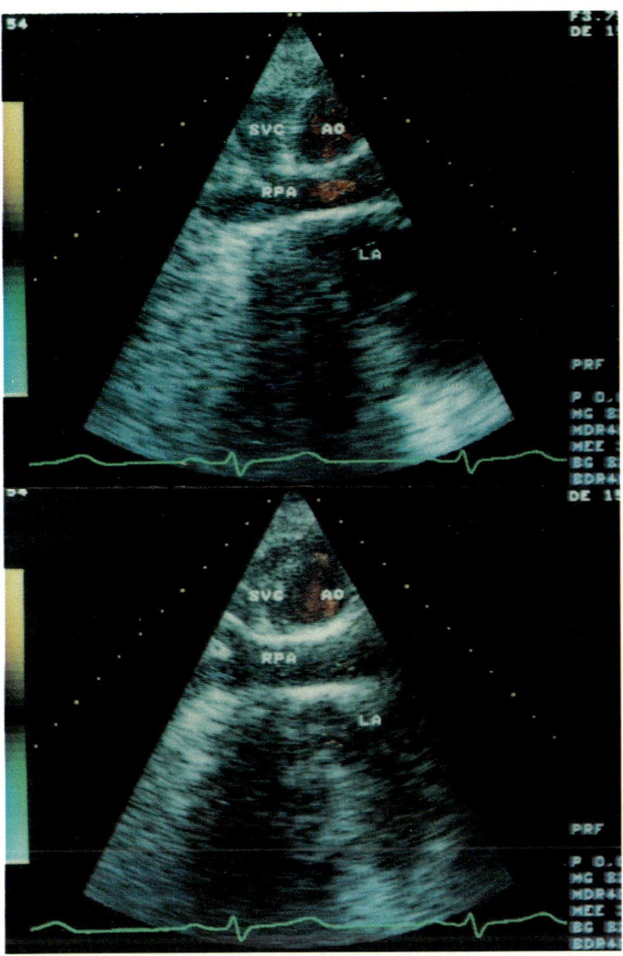

FIGURE 2-7—*Normal right pulmonary artery. Upper panel: with the transducer in the suprasternal notch, the right pulmonary artery is imaged along its length inferior to the transverse aorta. At points in the right pulmonary artery, flow is proceeding slightly away from the transducer, giving a blue signal. Where flow is roughly perpendicular to the path of the ultrasound, frequency dispersion is noted. The strong red signal in the proximal right pulmonary artery represents overlapping ascending aorta signal. Minimal posterior change in orientation of the transducer (lower panel) causes the artifactual flow signal in the right pulmonary artery to disappear. A small amount of frequency dispersion coding persists. Ao = aorta; LA = left atrium; RPA = right pulmonary artery; SVC = superior vena cava.*

normal, a blue signal is seen in the right pulmonary artery during systole with marked frequency dispersion if flow is rapid and the artery is nearly perpendicular to the imaging plane. Because the blood is travelling at a substantial angle to the path of ultrasound, the apparent velocity of blood in the right pulmonary artery is relatively low. Therefore, aliasing is highly unusual and absence of a signal may occur if flow is perpendicular to the path of the ultrasound. There is little or no color flow signal originating from the right pulmonary artery in diastole in normal individuals.

No matter where the transducer is placed on the surface of the body, the pulmonary veins always lie at a substantial distance. In the normal they carry blood at low velocities at a considerable angle of incidence to the ultrasonic path. Because of all these factors, the detection of pulmonary venous flow by color Doppler is inconsistent. Use of intensity function mapping rather than velocity mapping allows easier detection of pulmonary venous flow. Flow in the pulmonary veins can be detected with the transducer in the apical and subcostal positions (Figure 2-2). Flow generally occurs toward the transducer and is seen as a red signal in these views. Although phasic variation in velocity can produce an intermittently detectable signal on a velocity mapping system, there should be no sustained flow reversal in the pulmonary veins.

The color flow map in the left atrium is a composite of pulmonary venous inflow occurring continuously during the cardiac cycle and left atrial outflow during diastole across the mitral valve. In the normal there should be no signal of blood flow entering the left atrium across the atrial septum from the right atrium.

The color flow map of the normal left ventricle can be considered in two parts—the diastolic inflow of blood from the left atrium across the mitral valve and the systolic outflow of blood across the aortic valve to the aorta. From the apical transducer position, left ventricular inflow during diastole occurs centrally in the ventricle toward the transducer. Along the lateral and septal walls of the left ventricle, flow reversal may be a prominent feature of filling in late diastole (Figure 2-8). During early diastole the red signal which indicates blood flow toward the transducer is punctuated with blue, indicating rapid blood flow and aliasing. There is often some frequency dispersion during rapid filling in the normal. During mid-diastole, aliasing disappears as left ventricular inflow slows. In some normal individuals in late diastole, the increase in left ventricular inflow velocity brought about by atrial contraction will once again produce aliasing of the color flow map. The normal left ventricle does not receive significant inflow from any source other than the left atrium. Accordingly, there should be little or no flow signal in diastole in the subaortic region imaged from the apical and left parasternal positions (see Chapter 4). During systole, the left ventricle ejects blood across the aortic valve, and this can be demonstrated with color flow mapping with the transducer in the apical position (Figure 2-9). A blue signal indicating flow away from the transducer is noted from the ventricular apex to the aortic valve. There is some frequency dispersion within this signal and the blood flow can be fast enough

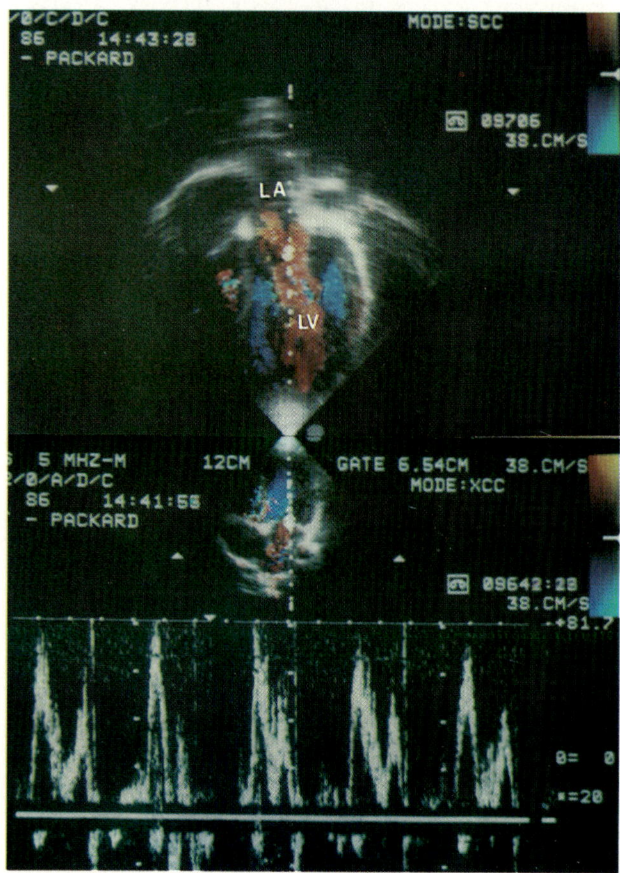

FIGURE 2-8—*Normal left ventricular inflow. The transducer is at the cardiac apex with the plane of ultrasound oriented to show a four-chamber view. A late diastolic frame with standard velocity and variance coding (upper panel) shows a red signal from left ventricular inflow with a small blue area due to aliasing. Note also the yellow speckles indicating frequency dispersion. Along the septal and lateral left ventricular walls there are blue signals indicating flow away from the transducer. This organized pattern of flow reversal during filling is normal; however, more complex and chaotic swirling may be seen in enlarged ventricles with poor function (see Chapter 9). The lower panel displays the corresponding pulsed Doppler tracing at the level of the mitral valve anulus. LA = left atrium; LV = left ventricle.*

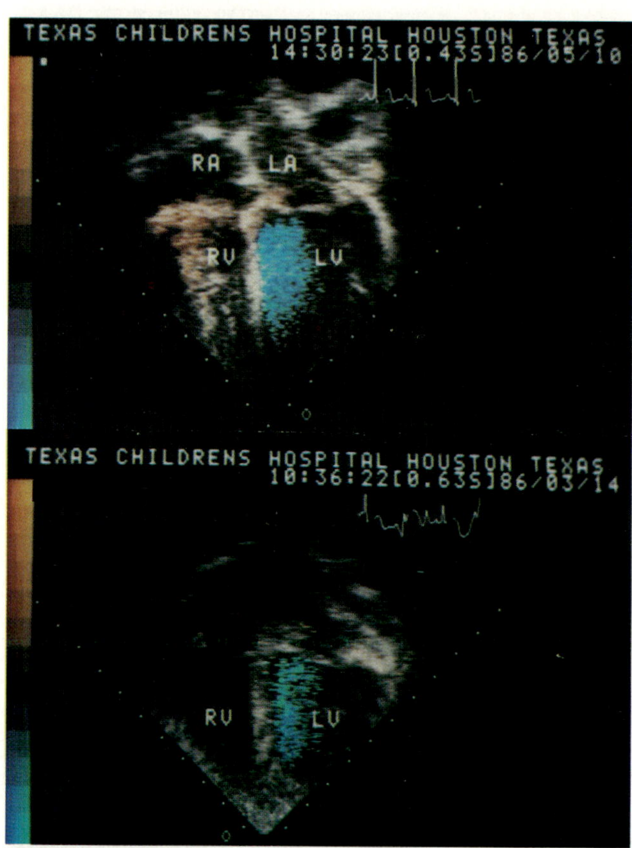

FIGURE 2-9—*Normal left ventricular outflow. With the transducer at the cardiac apex and the plane of the ultrasound directed slightly anterior to a standard four-chamber view, the blue signal from blood being ejected from the left ventricle is seen. LA = left atrium; LV = left ventricle; RA = right atrium; RV = right ventricle.*

in the normal to produce aliasing. Because the direction of blood flow in the left ventricular outflow tract is slightly toward the transducer in the parasternal long-axis view, a red signal may appear on the color Doppler display.

The color Doppler echocardiogram of the ascending aorta is best obtained from the suprasternal notch or high right parasternal transducer position. A strong red signal indicating flow toward the transducer in systole is normal (Figure 2-10). High-velocity flow with aliasing during systole in the ascending aorta is the rule (note blue within the red flow signal in Figure 2-10). Modest amounts of frequency dispersion during systole in the ascending aorta are normal; gross amounts of variance, however, are abnormal and suggest left ventricular outflow obstruction (see Chapter 3). A small amount of flow reversal in very early diastole in the ascending aorta can be seen in the normal; however, there is little or no color flow signal in the ascending aorta during most of diastole. Flow in the transverse aortic arch proceeds roughly perpendicular to the path of the ultrasound from the suprasternal notch. Therefore, a consistent color flow pattern in the transverse arch is uncommon. Blood flow at aortic branch points such as the origins of the innominate artery, left common carotid artery, and left subclavian artery may produce a very turbulent signal (often aliased) during systole on the color flow map (Figure 2-11).

Descending aortic flow is relatively fast away from the suprasternal notch or left infraclavicular transducer position. Normal descending aortic flow velocity is seen as a blue signal with red aliasing near the inner curvature during systole (Figure 2-12). There is little or no signal

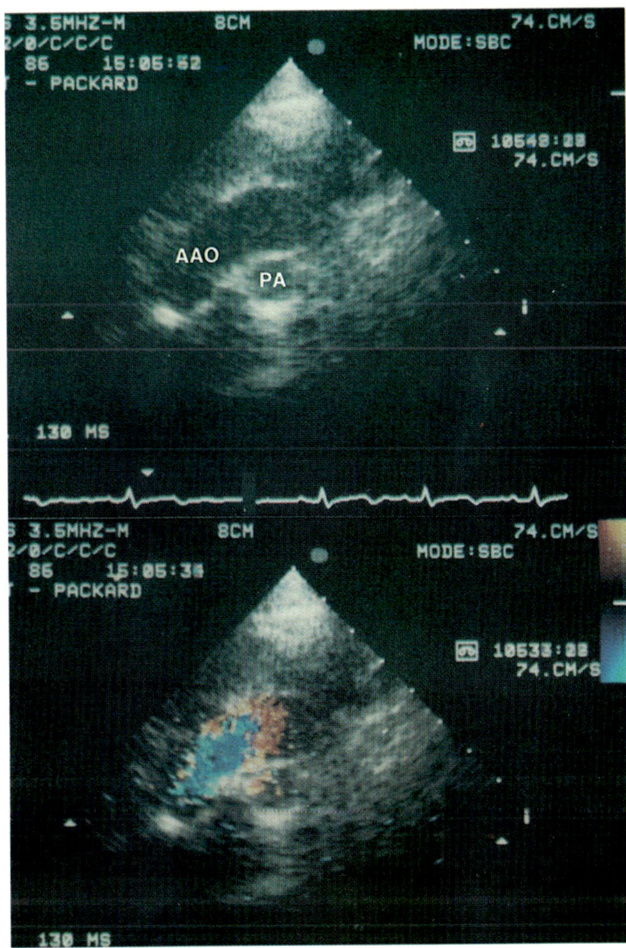

FIGURE 2-10—*Normal ascending aorta. With the transducer in the suprasternal notch, ascending aortic flow toward the transducer is rapid enough to produce a very prominent alias blue within the red signal. This was recorded without variance coding. Considerable variance may be seen in the ascending aorta (AAO), particularly along the walls and as it approaches the transverse aortic arch (compare with Figure 2-11). PA = pulmonary artery.*

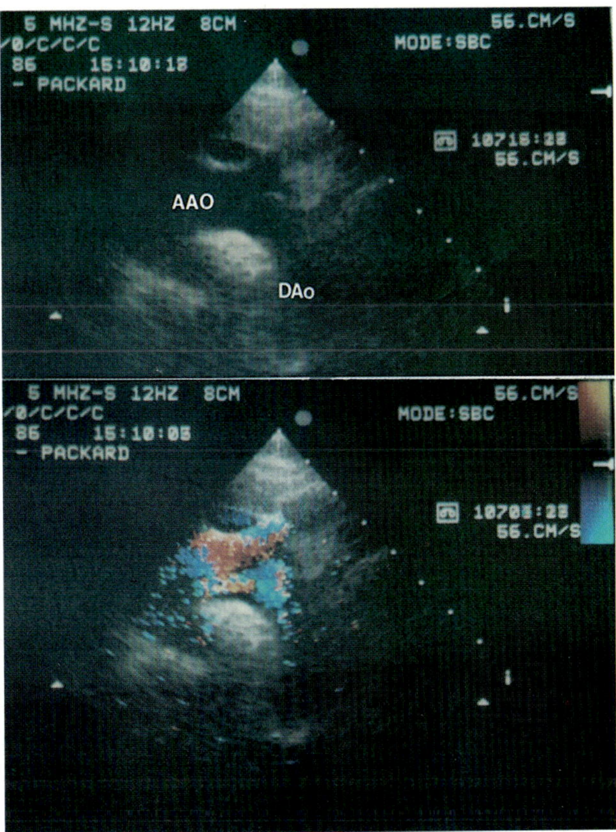

FIGURE 2-11—*Normal aorta. Upper panel: the distal ascending aorta (AAO) and the transverse aortic arch are imaged from the suprasternal notch. Lower panel: branch points of aortic arch are associated with high-velocity flow and frequency dispersion in the normal. Shown here is the origin of the innominate artery. DAo = descending aorta.*

from the descending aorta throughout most of diastole (see Chapter 10). It is often possible to image the distal thoracic and abdominal aorta from the subcostal transducer position such that blood flow is directed somewhat toward the transducer. With the transducer lower on the abdomen and directed more posteriorly, the abdominal aorta can be imaged as in Figure 2-3 (lower panel). An inconsistent signal is usual because in portions of the abdominal aorta, flow will be directly perpendicular to the path of the ultrasound and will not produce a flow map. In other parts of the abdominal aorta, the flow produces a red or blue signal, depending on the orientation of the aorta relative to the transducer. This is another situation in which the blood flow is close to perpendicular to the path of the ultrasound, so its apparent velocity is relatively slow.

It should be obvious at this point that the normal color Doppler examination is unfortunately not a single picture. It is instead a composite of many individual normal segments. Each normal segment, in turn, is a composite of a number of normal flow velocity maps at differing times in the cardiac cycle. The echocardiographer performing color Doppler must therefore synthesize all the individual parts of the color Doppler examination into a meaningful whole. Recognition of clinically significant abnormalities of the color Doppler display depends on the completeness of the examination and the confidence with which the echocardiographer recognizes the normal color Doppler findings.

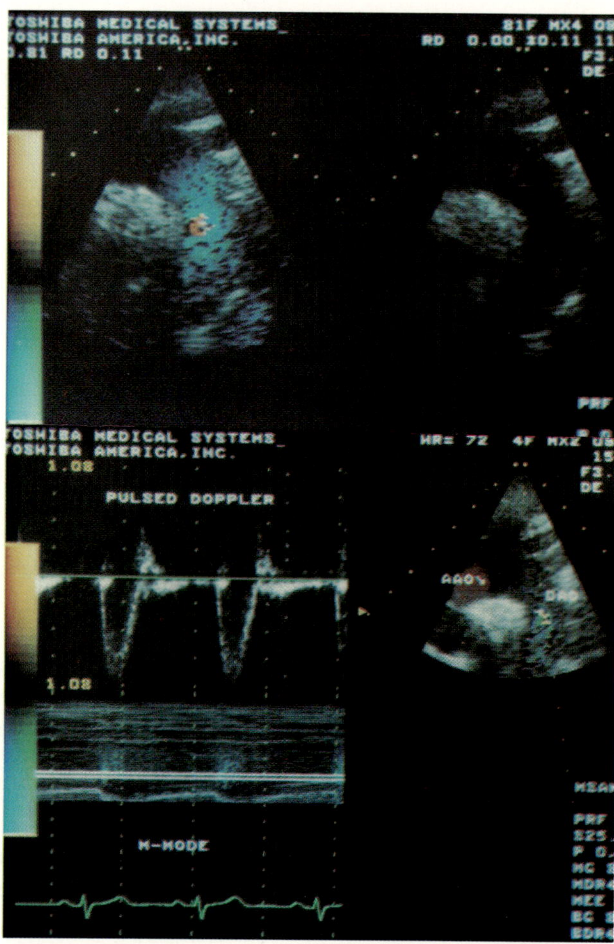

FIGURE 2-12—*Normal upper descending aorta. With the transducer in the suprasternal notch, color Doppler shows the flow pattern in the normal descending aorta (DAo). A blue signal (upper panel) demonstrates flow velocity away from the transducer with regional aliasing (red) in the aortic isthmus. The lower panel shows the corresponding pulsed Doppler recording from the descending aorta. Note the transient flow reversal at end of systole which might be apparent in some normal color Doppler recordings gated to that point in the cardiac cycle. AAo = ascending aorta; DAo = descending aorta.*

References

1. Switzer DF, Nanda NC: Doppler color flow mapping. Ultrasound Med Biol 3:403-416, 1985.
2. Sahn DJ: Real-time two-dimensional Doppler echocardiographic flow mapping. Circulation 71:849-853, 1985.
3. Schoenfeld MR: Focus on: Color-coded, real-time, two-dimensional Doppler echocardiographic mapping of intracardiac blood flow. J Cardiovasc Ultrasonography 4:3-4, 1985.
4. Omoto R: Color Atlas of Real-Time Two Dimensional Doppler Echocardiography. Tokyo, Sinden-To-Chiryosha, 1983.
5. Nimura Y, Miyatake K: Recent progress in ultrasonic diagnosis of the heart: Doppler flow imaging. Jpn Circ J 49:694-701, 1985.
6. Miyatake K, Shiro I, Shimizu A, et al: Right atrial flow topography in healthy subjects studied with real-time two-dimensional Doppler flow imaging techniques. J Am Coll Cardiol 7:425-431, 1986.
7. Recusani F, Valdes-Cruz L, Dalton N, et al: Tricuspid and pulmonary insufficiency and right heart flow patterns in normals: Studies using color coded flow mapping and pulsed Doppler. Circulation 72(Suppl III):III-307, 1985 (abstr).

Chapter 3

Stenotic Lesions

Achi Ludomirsky, M.D., and James C. Huhta, M.D.

Doppler methodology has provided a tremendous aid to two-dimensional echocardiographic imaging in a variety of congenital heart diseases, especially in valvular disorders.[1] Detecting the velocity across a stenotic valve often yields a quantitative assessment of the severity which otherwise requires cardiac catheterization. Doppler supplements two-dimensional imaging by prediction of the pressure gradient and in some cases can predict the valve area.[2]

The Doppler techniques that are used to evaluate valvular disorders are similar in both children and adults. The fluid dynamics of valvular stenosis have been well demonstrated using flow models and the limitations of very small orifice size have been estimated, but there is currently little clinical work in the presence of ventricular dysfunction. In the face of adequate function, the blood flow proximal to a discrete obstruction is laminar and normal in velocity and usually does not exceed one meter per second. In cases of obstructive lesions the velocity of blood flow in the obstructed orifice is increased, creating a high-velocity jet in which the blood flow remains laminar. Shortly after the obstructive area the jet extends downstream and the blood cells move in a different direction away from the center line. The blood cell velocity also decreases with progressive distance from the jet. This area of the flow disturbance immediately beyond the obstructive lesion generates a broad spectrum of nonlinear Doppler shifts. Distally, the velocity of the red blood cell returns to normal values and the blood flow again becomes laminar.[1]

In-vitro studies show that both pulsed and continuous-wave Doppler accurately predict the valvular pressure gradient at various cardiac outputs.[3,4] Clinical studies have shown that Doppler measurements of high velocities of flow through stenotic valves correlate with the degree of stenosis. Measuring the peak jet velocity (V_{max}) from the spectral display and using the modified Bernoulli equation (Pressure gradient $= 4 \times V_{max}^2$) has been used to estimate the peak instantaneous pressure gradient across the stenotic valve. It should be emphasized that the pressure differences measured by Doppler echocardiography represent peak instantaneous values and not peak- to-peak or mean pressure gradients. It is possible to measure the mean gradients by point-by-point conversion, then integration of the Doppler wave form taking into account the time lag introduced by fluid-filled catheters. Some limitations of this methodology should be noted. First, desirable spectral display data cannot be recorded in all patients. Second, the maximum instantaneous pressure difference usually exceeds the peak-to-peak pressure gradient at catheterization, especially in left ventricular outflow obstruction. And third, the volume of the flow through the stenotic valve has an important influence on the pressure gradient. In a child or adult with low cardiac output and poor ventricular function, it is possible to underestimate the severity of obstruction.[5] To overcome these limitations several investigators used pulsed Doppler techniques for quantitative evaluation of flow disturbances beyond the stenotic valve.[6] They showed differences between mild, moderate, and severe degrees of obstruction based on the flow diameters.

Color Doppler is a two-dimensional display of intracardiac flow velocities. It is a pulsed Doppler technique that has the advantage of depth accuity and the disadvantage of the inability to quantitate high velocities. In stenotic lesions color Doppler aids in (1) visualization of the jet color, (2) detection of the presence of multiple jets, and (3) assessment of the jet direction across the stenotic valve. By using directed continuous-wave Doppler in conjunction with color Doppler, the maximum velocity of the jet can be obtained.

Aortic Stenosis

Two-dimensional echocardiography can be used to characterize the lesions that produce left ventricular outflow tract obstruction. These include valvular aortic stenosis, discrete subaortic stenosis, hypertrophic obstructive cardiomyopathy and supravalvular aortic stenosis. Two-dimensional echocardiography can visualize the centrally located aortic valve and valvular abnormalities are readily detected. The thickening of the aortic valve is particularly evident during diastole. The severity of the stenosis is best appreciated during systole when the dome shape of the valve with the restricted opening is visualized. The diameter of this opening approximates the severity of the stenosis.[1] Imaging of the ascending aorta shows a widening of the lumen superior to the valve as a result of poststenotic dilatation.

Doppler is useful in measuring the degree of obstruction to left ventricular ejection.[7,8] Although no single view is ideal, the systolic jet of aortic stenosis may be detected from a variety of echocardiographic views using continuous-wave Doppler. Color flow mapping supplements pulsed and continuous-wave Doppler in determining the site of obstruction. In general, the color Doppler flow imaging examination of the stenotic aortic valve will show a narrow band of flow emitted from a restrictive valve orifice seen as a blue jet entering the aortic root although aliasing begins well below the valve with significant obstruction.[4] Aliasing is seen as a red area and turbulence as a mosaic pattern once the velocity of red blood cells exceeds the peak repetition frequency at that depth (see Chapter 1). The diameter of the origin of the jet is roughly inversely proportional to the severity of the stenosis. The actual pressure gradient can be determined using the continuous-wave Doppler aligned to the stenotic jet identified by color Doppler. The position

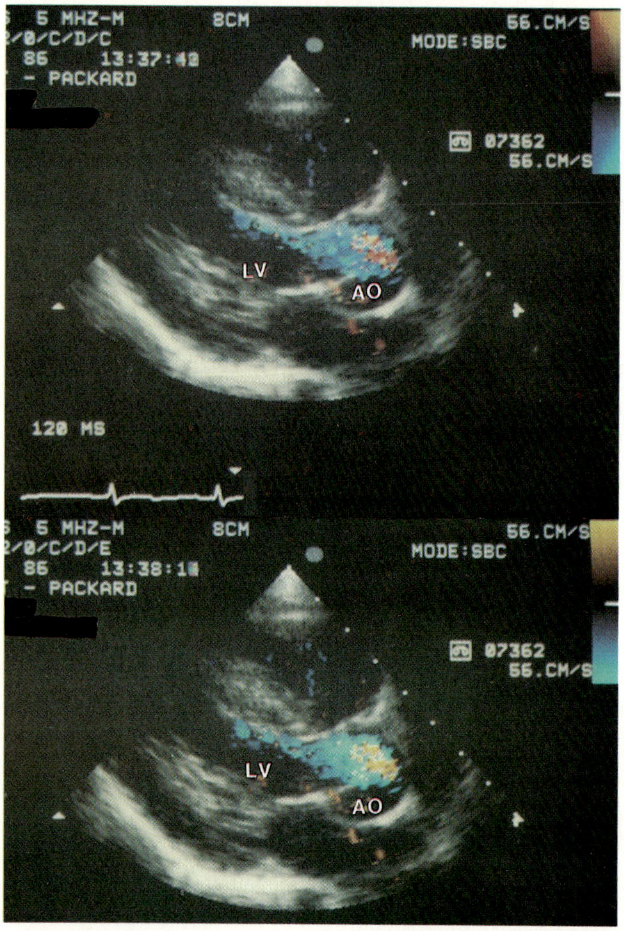

FIGURE 3-1—*Parasternal scan in a patient with bicuspid aortic valve and mild aortic stenosis. Two modes of Doppler display are used on the same information—with (upper panel) and without variance (lower panel). The blue jet arising from the left ventricular outflow tract entering the aortic root aliases distal to the obstruction and the mosaic jet is eccentric. Ao = aorta; LV = left ventricle.*

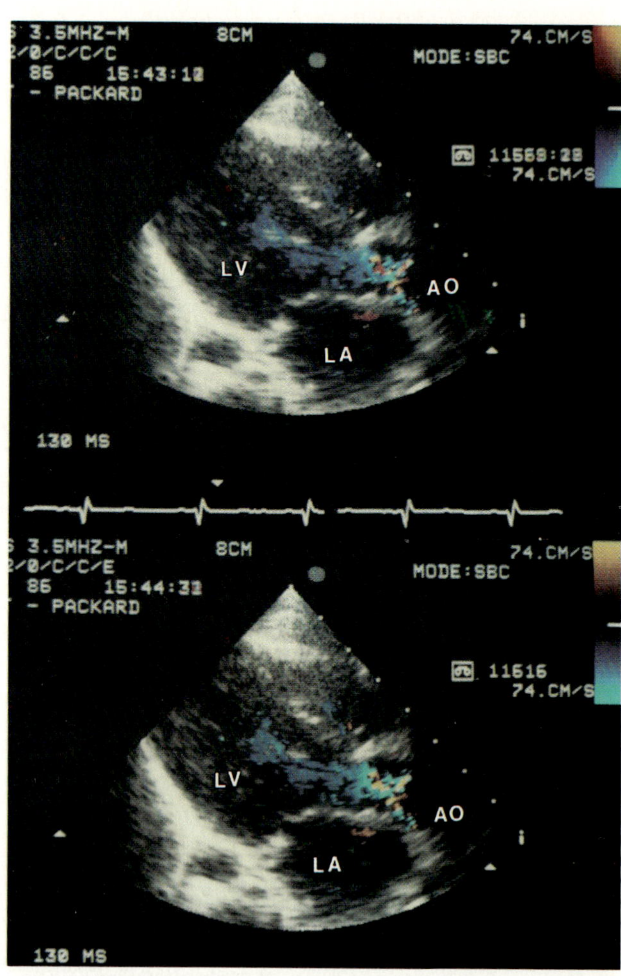

FIGURE 3-2—*Parasternal long-axis view of a patient with mild aortic stenosis in which continuous-wave Doppler predicted the gradient to be 35 mmHg. The mosaic pattern indicating turbulence and impairment of laminar flow localized the obstruction to the valve area (variance display in the upper panel) on a frame gated to systole (130 milliseconds after the r wave of the electrocardiogram). Display without variance is included for comparison (lower panel). Obstruction in the subvalve area or the left ventricular outflow tract is excluded. AO = aorta; LA = left atrium; LV = left ventricle.*

from which the highest velocity can be recorded in children and young adults may be the suprasternal notch, the first or second right intercostal space, or the apical position. Occasional patients with aortic valve stenosis may also have an increased velocity in the left ventricular outflow tract that indicates obstruction with moderate pressure drops proximal to the valve. Some of these patients have additional dynamic narrowing of the left ventricular outflow tract due to hypertrophy. Color flow mapping facilitates the visualization of the high-velocity jet and variance denotes the site of peak velocities whether they occur in the left ventricular outflow tract or the aortic valvular or supravalvular regions.

The most common form of congenital heart defect is bicuspid aortic valve which usually leads to significant aortic stenosis in later life. In childhood the murmur and ejection click can be detected and echocardiographic examination confirms the eccentricity of the valve and its opening pattern. Color Doppler can also be used to display graphically this eccentricity (Figure 3-1). The site of the obstruction at the valve is confirmed by the color display (Figure 3-2). The shape of the resulting jet in the ascending aorta depends on the details of the valvular abnormality but the jet direction is usually anterior and to the right (Figure 3-3). Transmission of turbulence into the aorta and aortic arch is better appreciated by color Doppler than in any other way (Figure 3-4).

In the presence of *subaortic stenosis*, a color Doppler variance display will indicate the mosaic pattern proximal to the valve in the left ventricular outflow tract area (Figures 3-5 and 3-6). The jet that is normally depicted blue indicating flow away from the transducer will turn to a mosaic pattern about 1 to 2 cm below the valve area. The visualization of the high-velocity mosaic

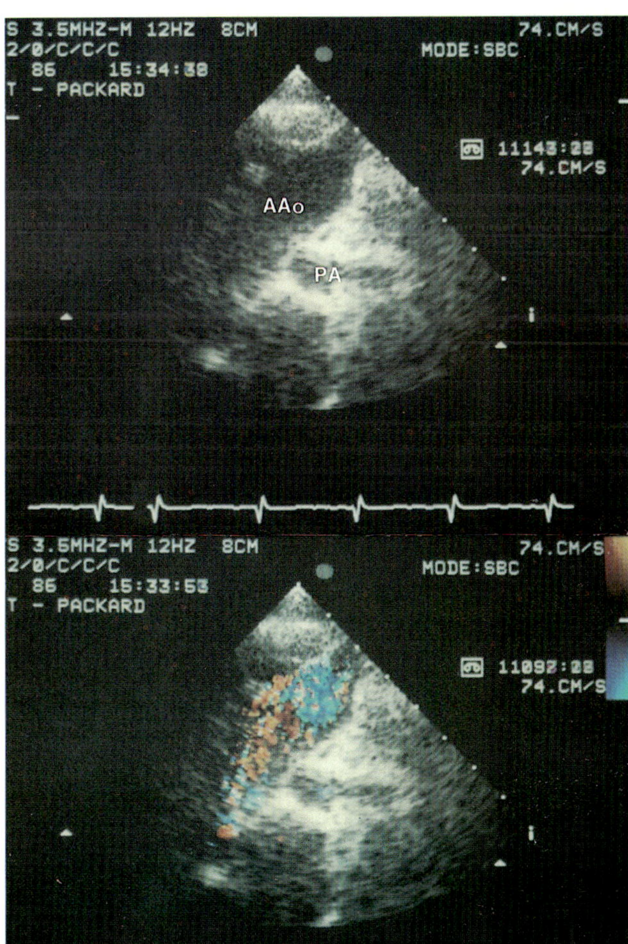

FIGURE 3-3—*Suprasternal view of a two-year-old with severe aortic stenosis. The color display in this case shows a triangular jet arising from the aortic valve into the ascending aorta (AAo) in a mosaic pattern indicating turbulence. PA = pulmonary artery.*

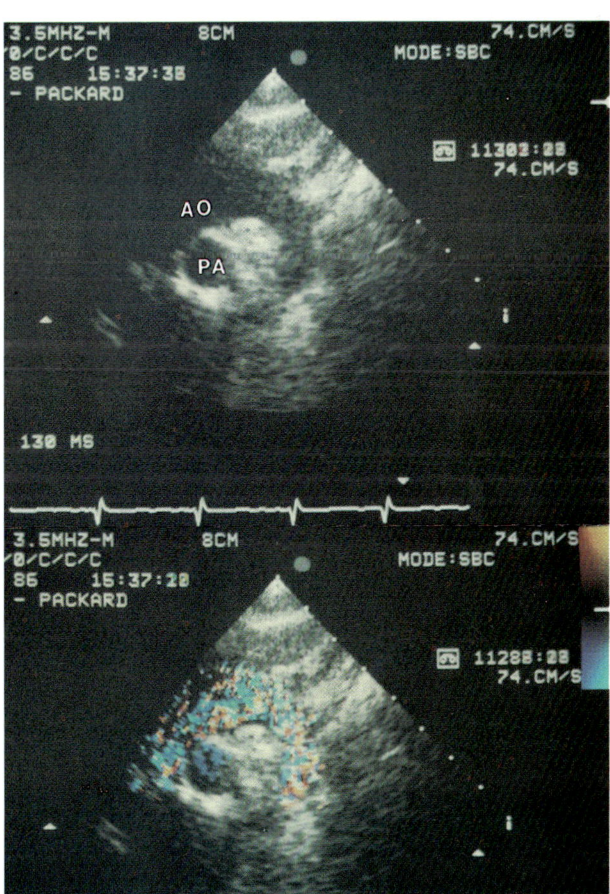

FIGURE 3-4—*Evaluation of the aortic arch (AO) using suprasternal scans revealed turbulence that reached the transverse aortic arch and the descending aorta in aortic valve stenosis. Continuous-wave Doppler confirmed the diagnosis of severe aortic stenosis with 120 mmHg gradient across the valve. The extent of turbulence in this vessel depends on the severity of the stenosis but also on the myocardial function. PA = right pulmonary artery.*

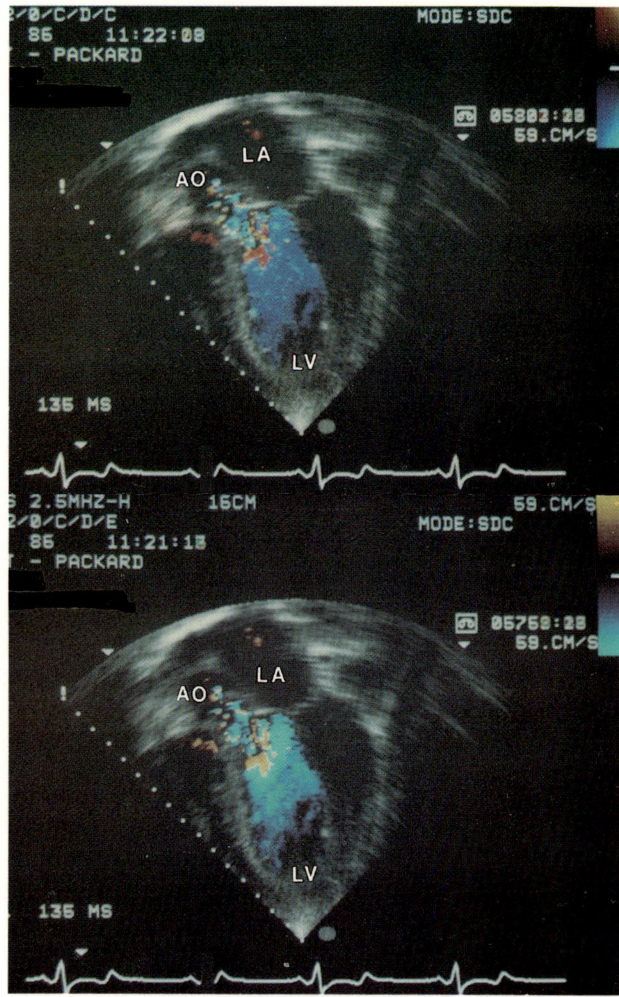

FIGURE 3-5—*Apical long-axis view of a patient with mild aortic valve stenosis and trivial subaortic stenosis. This is an important view in the evaluation of aortic stenosis for the detection of left ventricular outflow tract obstruction but valvular and subvalvular obstruction cannot be differentiated on this frame. Variance (upper panel) and nonvariance display (lower panel) give similar information. AO = aorta; LA = left atrium; LV = left ventricle.*

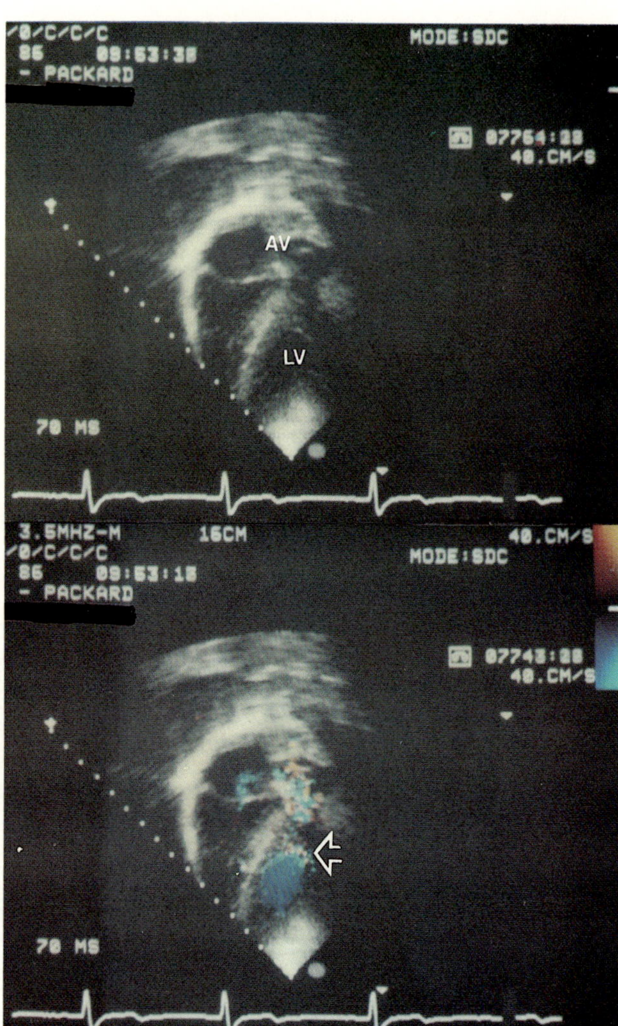

FIGURE 3-6—*Apical long-axis scan in a ten-year-old girl with discrete subaortic stenosis showing variance in the subaortic region (open white arrow in the lower panel) below the aortic valve (AV). LV = left ventricle.*

jet assists the alignment of the continuous-wave Doppler beam for accurate assessment of peak velocities (Figure 3-7).

There is a great importance of timing during the cardiac cycle in the evaluation of aortic stenosis. Figure 3-8 is a modified apical four-chamber view showing the color pattern during the very beginning of the ejection and shortly after the opening of the aortic valve. The differentiation between the high-velocity jet produced by aortic stenosis and that produced by other lesions is important and it is useful to use the color Doppler display by gating with the electrocardiogram. Color Doppler can differentiate two systolic jets, such as aortic stenosis and mitral regurgitation, which may be confused using continuous-wave Doppler only (Figures 3-8 and 3-9). Gating allows the examiner to concentrate on one portion of the cardiac cycle which can be difficult at higher heart rates found in children and infants. Because of the often hyperdynamic ventricular function, there is often variance under the aortic valve in infants with aortic valve stenosis (Figure 3-10). A maximum velocity greater than 2.5 meters per second suggests mild obstruction in the absence of anemia with normal ventricular function.

Supravalvular aortic stenosis can be difficult to diagnose and color Doppler screening may not show the jet if the angle with the lesion is not optimal (Figure 3-11).

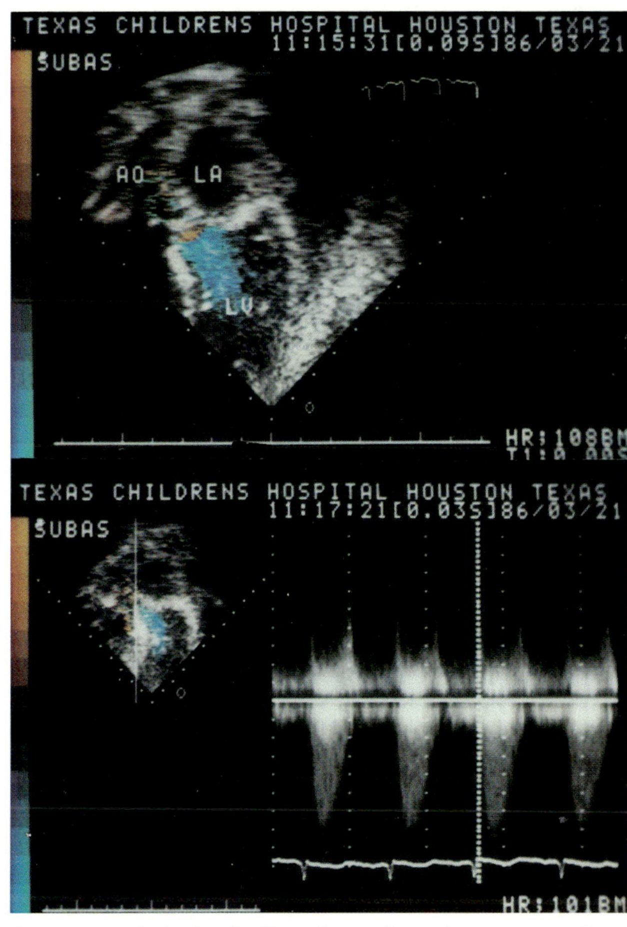

FIGURE 3-7—*Apical color Doppler and continuous-wave Doppler in mild-moderate subaortic stenosis with a velocity of 3.5 meters per second corresponding to a gradient of 50 mmHg. Note the imperfect alignment of the continuous-wave Doppler line with the left ventricular outflow tract (lower panel). AO = aorta; LA = left atrium; LV = left ventricle.*

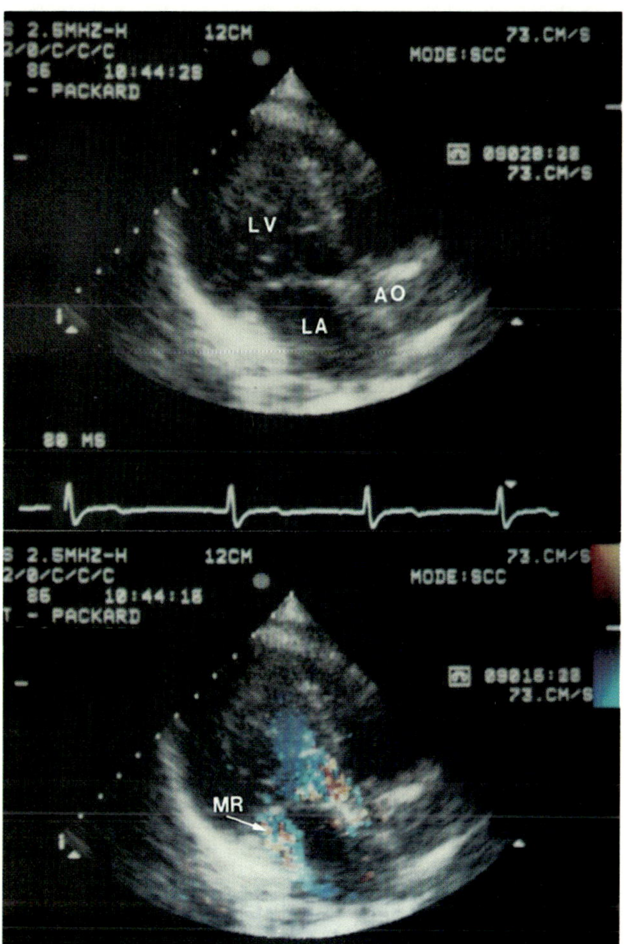

FIGURE 3-8—*Apical long-axis scan of subaortic stenosis in an 11-year-old boy. The pattern of ejection at the onset of systole (lower panel) illustrates the change in velocity pattern (mosaic) during ejection. Note the presence of additional mitral regurgitation (MR) on color Doppler (lower panel and Figure 3-9). AO = aorta; LA = left atrium; LV = left ventricle.*

Suprasternal scans with color Doppler should detect the flow disturbance (Figure 3-4). Dynamic subaortic stenosis in hypertrophic cardiomyopathy is discussed in Chapter 9.

In summary, color Doppler in aortic stenosis provides three kinds of information about this hemodynamic abnormality. First is the direction of the flow, second the speed, and third the resulting turbulence. Combining these three factors helps in the comprehension of the picture of blood flow through the stenotic lesion. Accurate localization of the level of stenosis throughout the left ventricular outflow tract is easily achieved and directed continuous wave can be aligned with the jet direction in two planes.

Pulmonary Valve Stenosis

The most common cause of right ventricular outflow obstruction in children is valvular pulmonary stenosis. Severe pulmonary valve stenosis causing symptoms of cardiac failure in the first month of life can be diagnosed by noninvasive techniques. The two-dimensional echocardiogram will reveal the right ventricular hypertrophy and the abnormal pulmonary valve. The parasternal short-axis view at the level of the great artery reveals a well-developed pulmonary artery with poststenotic dilatation. Usually the closed pulmonary valve produces a dense echo shadow indicative of a thickened valve. In mild to moderate pulmonary valve

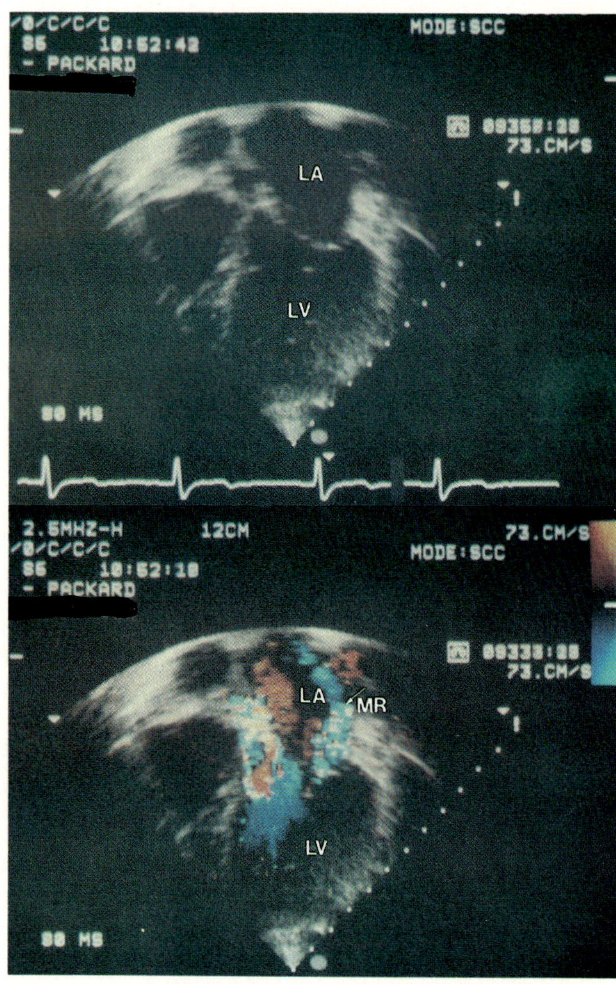

FIGURE 3-9—*Apical view of aortic stenosis and mitral regurgitation in systole. Abbreviations as in Figure 3-8.*

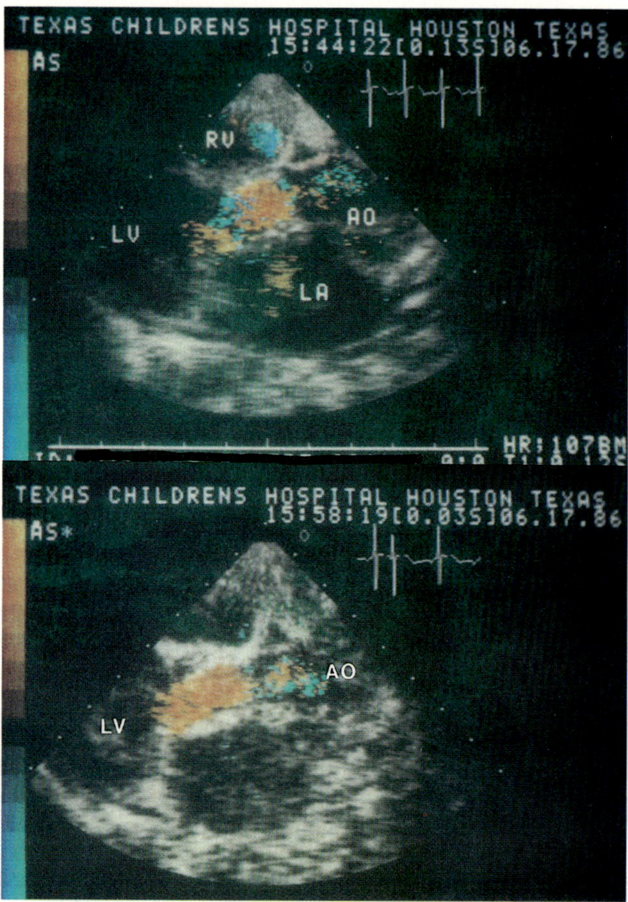

FIGURE 3-10—*Parasternal view of aortic valve stenosis in an infant. Note the mosaic pattern above the valve and the transition zone of color Doppler velocity findings at the valve. AO = aorta; LA = left atrium; LV = left ventricle; RV = right ventricle.*

stenosis, the two- dimensional echocardiography may be of little or no diagnostic value because the abnormality of the pulmonary valve and the right ventricular hypertrophy may be difficult to recognize.

Doppler techniques are useful for the evaluation of the gradient in pulmonary stenosis and accurately predict the instantaneous and peak-to-peak gradients. The subcostal view aiming toward the right ventricular outflow tract is a useful window for evaluation of the pulmonary valve with Doppler and usually gives the highest gradients. Jet velocities can usually be recorded with the transducer in the second or third left intercostal space directed posteriorly, and superiorly.[10]

Color Doppler of the pulmonary valve area is useful for location of the level of obstruction, evaluation of the persistence of infundibular stenosis, and follow-up results of surgery and dilatation of the pulmonary valve (Figure 3-12). Subvalvular, supravalvular, or peripheral stenosis can be documented and the gradient can be estimated with continuous-wave Doppler using the modified Bernoulli equation (Figure 3-13). Subcostal views are useful if adequate imaging can be obtained (Figure 3-14).

Balloon dilatation of the pulmonary valve is the preferable modality for treatment of pulmonary valve stenosis in children. Color Doppler is of help in evaluating these patients noninvasively pre- and postdilatation (Figure 3-15). The dynamic nature of infundibular obstruction and its course after dilation can be followed. Increased velocity in the pulmonary artery is also seen with increased flow as with a significant left-to-right shunt or with significant pulmonary regurgitation, but

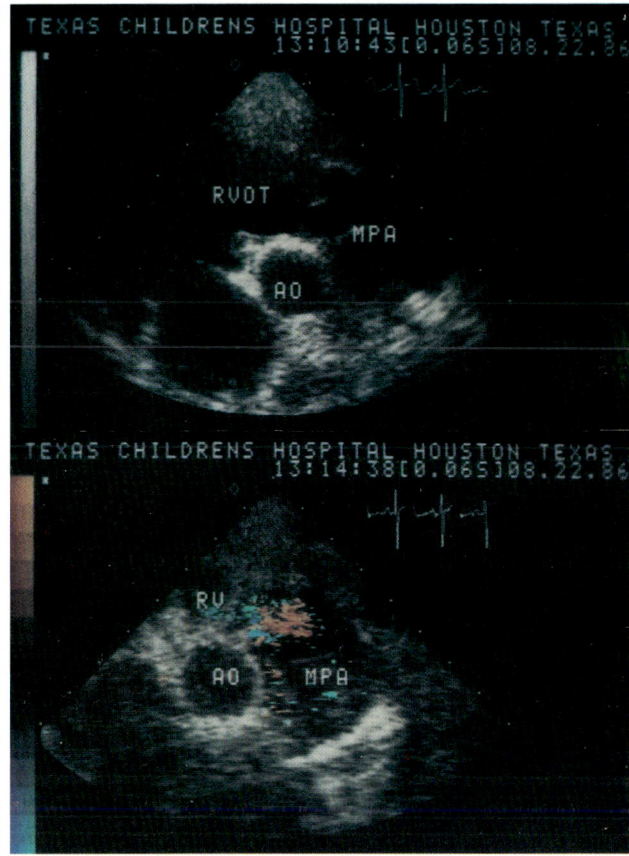

FIGURE 3-11—*Parasternal long-axis view of supravalvular aortic stenosis (white arrow in the upper panel) in a seven-year-old boy. Note the mosaic pattern in the left ventricular outflow tract but poor sensitivity to the presence of obstruction above the valve. AO = aorta; AV = aortic valve; LA = left atrium; LV = left ventricle; RV = right ventricle.*

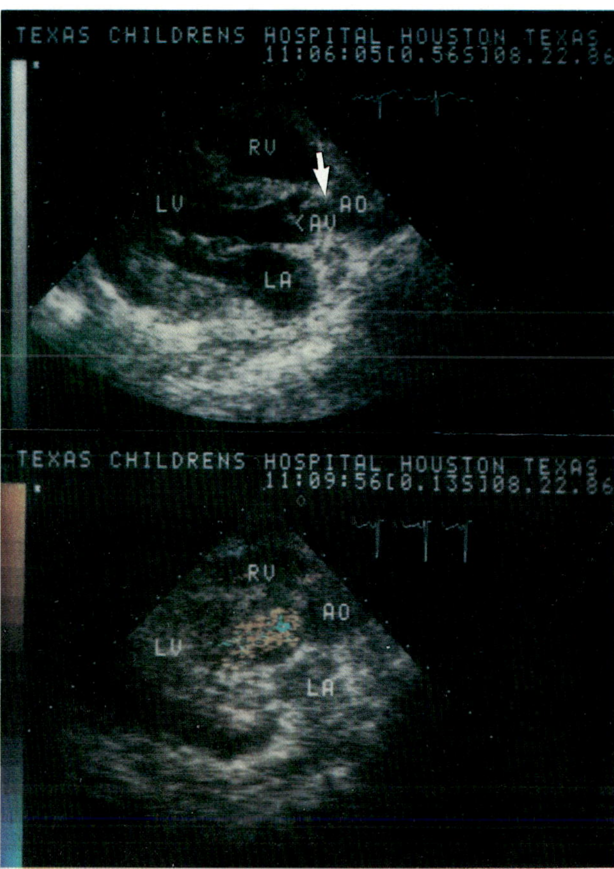

FIGURE 3-12—*Parasternal short-axis view of a patient with mild pulmonary valve stenosis. The lower panel depicts a jet directed from the right ventricular outflow tract (RVOT) toward the main pulmonary artery (MPA). Aliasing of the blue jet occurs at the level of the valve cusps and the red jet surrounded by a vortex of blue jet indicates that a high velocity is present. Note the poststenotic dilatation of the MPA. AO = aorta.*

these findings rarely exceed 2 meters per second. Figures 3-16 and 3-17 illustrate this in a color Doppler examination of a five-year-old boy with absent pulmonary valve syndrome, a condition where the valve tissue is undeveloped.

Color Doppler is useful in the detection of peripheral pulmonary stenosis. Using high parasternal scans, the layered pattern in the main pulmonary artery can be appreciated using gated frames in systole (Figure 3-18).

In conclusion, color Doppler in pulmonary stenosis is useful for the detection of the jet and for more accurate prediction of the valve gradient. The location of the obstruction, particularly if dynamic, can be suspected and serial noninvasive follow-up in patients after surgical or dilatation treatment can be performed.

Mitral Stenosis

In mitral stenosis the pressure drop calculated from the noninvasive Doppler recordings of maximal velocity in the mitral jet correlates well with pressure recordings at catheterization. Velocity of mitral flow is usually best recorded from the apical area with the transducer directed posteriorly and slightly superiorly. Continuous-wave Doppler is best for the determination of the pressure gradient across the mitral valve from the left atrium to the left ventricle.[11] The peak instantaneous pressure gradient could be measured by the modified Bernoulli equation; gradient is equal to $4\ V^2$. The mean gradient can be calculated by measuring the area under the curve of the instantaneous $4\ V^2$ gradient versus time. Using the pressure half-time can yield more accurate measure-

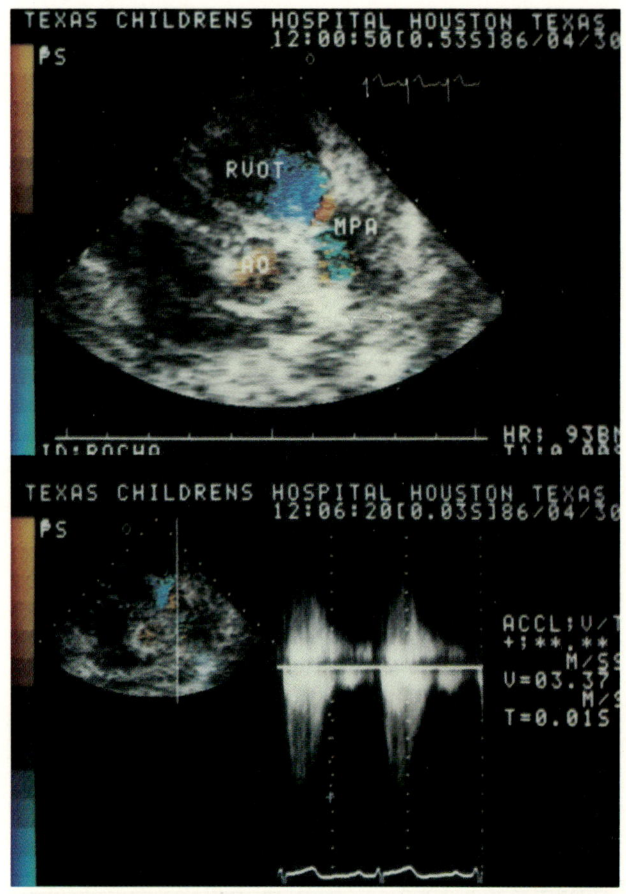

FIGURE 3-13—*Short-axis parasternal view of a patient with moderate pulmonary valve stenosis. The upper panel depicts a blue jet away from the transducer from the right ventricular outflow tract (RVOT) toward the main pulmonary artery. There is a wide blue jet in the area of the right ventricular outflow tract with aliasing just proximal to the valve. Distal to the valve there is a narrow mosaic pattern indicating high velocity in the main pulmonary artery. Directed continuous-wave Doppler aligned parallel to the jet in the main pulmonary artery showed a peak velocity of 3.4 meters per second.*

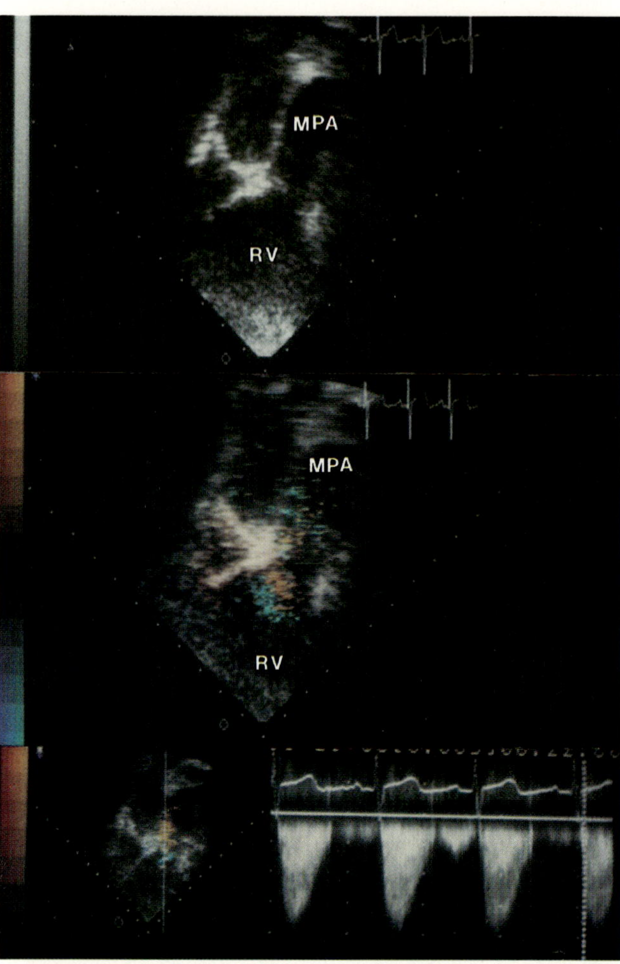

FIGURE 3-14—*A three-year-old child with mild pulmonary stenosis. A subcostal view of the right ventricular outflow tract shows aliasing starting proximal to the valve and a mosaic pattern indicating high velocity is shown in the main pulmonary artery (middle panel). The lower panel shows the spectral display of the continuous-wave Doppler using the jet as a guide to sampling in the right ventricular outflow tract.*

ment of the mitral valve area[12] and has the advantage of being less sensitive to altered cardiac output. The effective mitral valve area (cm^2) can be approximated by the formula that the mitral valve area is equal to 220 divided by the pressure half-time (milliseconds). A reliable estimate of the mitral valve area from the maximal mitral flow velocity curve is possible. This method is especially useful in patients with associated mitral regurgitation.[1]

Color Doppler provides information about the direction of the blood flow, its velocity, and the presence of turbulence. Khandheria and his associates at the Mayo Clinic carefully studied the visualization and the characterization of the blood flow jet in mitral stenosis.[13] In a report of 37 color Doppler studies, the appearance of the mitral stenotic jet was characterized in all patients. The typical jet has a candle flame appearance with a central blue zone due to an aliasing from a high velocity surrounded by a vortex of yellow-red representing turbulence toward the transducer. Although they visualized various jet configurations, most frequently the jets were

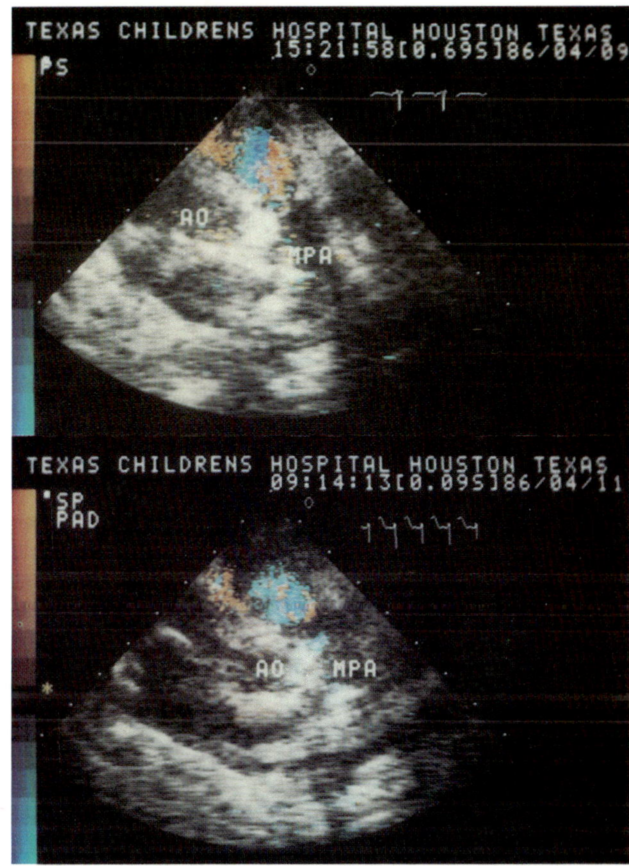

FIGURE 3-15—*High parasternal views of the right ventricular outflow tract before (upper panel) and after (lower panel) balloon valvuloplasty. Note the aliasing proximal to the valve which continues in a mosaic pattern toward the main pulmonary artery. In comparison, note the lack of mosaic pattern under the valve after dilation. AO = aorta; MPA = main pulmonary artery.*

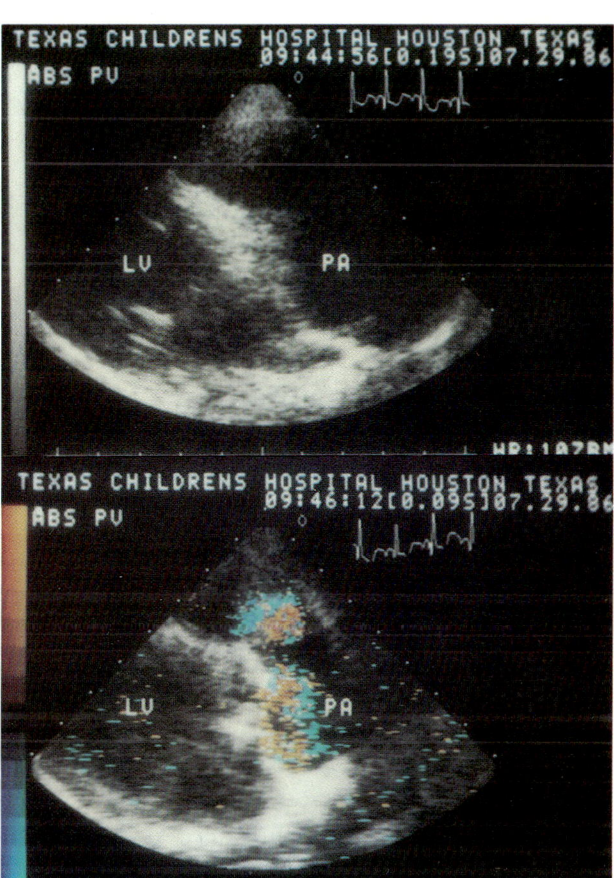

FIGURE 3-16—*Two-dimensional imaging from a short- axis parasternal view of absent pulmonary valve syndrome. Note the huge dilatation of the main pulmonary artery (PA). Color Doppler shows a systolic mosaic pattern in the main pulmonary artery just distal to the right ventricular outflow tract with pulmonary insufficiency.*

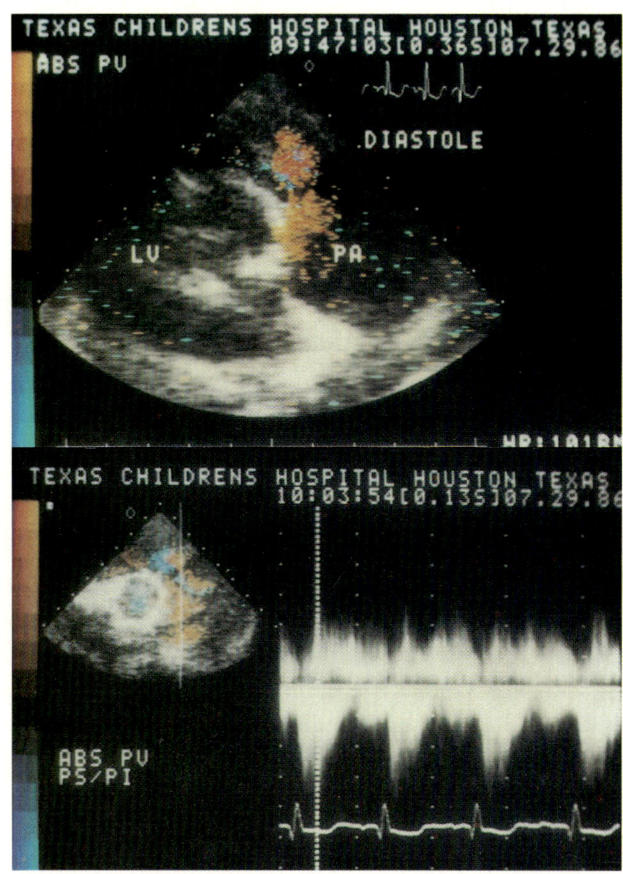

FIGURE 3-17—*Absent pulmonary valve syndrome in the same patient as in Figure 3-16. Diastole shows a red jet flow toward the transducer indicative of pulmonary insufficiency. In the lower panel is depicted the spectral display of the continuous-wave Doppler of this patient which shows a typical pattern of trivial pulmonary stenosis with pulmonary insufficiency.*

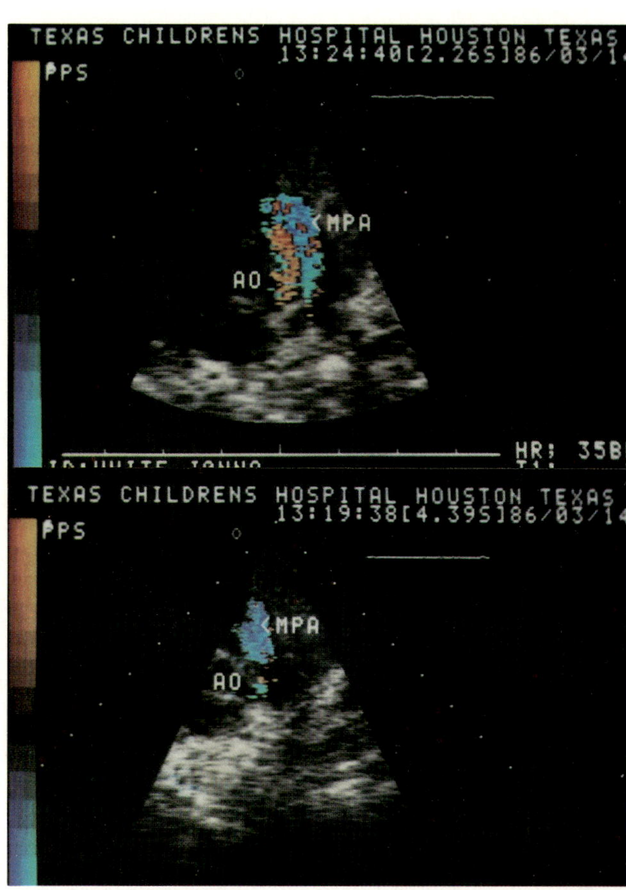

FIGURE 3-18—*Parasternal view of color Doppler in peripheral pulmonary stenosis. Aliasing occurs in systolic frames distal to the bifurcation of the main pulmonary artery (MPA) in the right pulmonary artery indicating peripheral stenosis in this area.*

centrally and apically directed. In 9 percent of their patients the jets were eccentric. They found that color Doppler visualization of the jet facilitated more accurate alignment of the continuous-wave Doppler and thereby enhanced the accuracy of the Doppler data that were obtained.

Congenital mitral stenosis is quite different anatomically from acquired disease. However, the same concepts can be applied to the hemodynamic assessment (Figures 3-19 and 3-20). Rheumatic mitral disease can occur in childhood and presents a pattern similar to that found in adults (Figure 3-21). Color Doppler also can be useful to detect supravalvular mitral ring (Figure 3-22), double

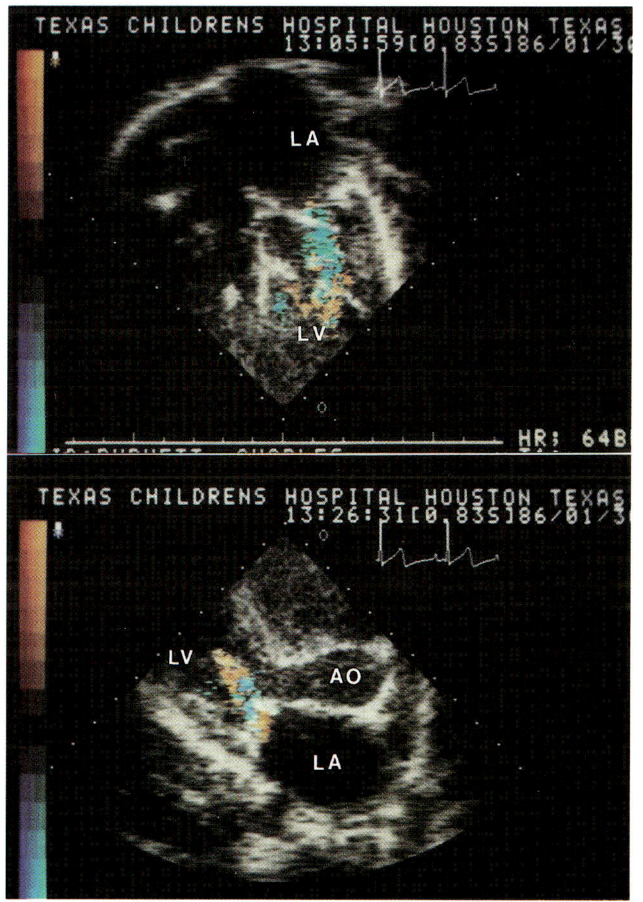

FIGURE 3-19—*Diastolic still frame of a five-year-old boy with congenital mitral stenosis. Apical four-chamber view shows a typical candle-like appearance of mitral stenosis in early diastole (upper panel). The inflow is restricted to a narrow band directed from the stenotic orifice. Aliasing results in the center of a jet where a blue zone is surrounded by a yellow vortex giving the appearance of the candlelight or flame. In the lower panel of the same patient, the parasternal long-axis view demonstrates the narrow band of flow arising from the left atrium toward the left ventricle. Note that the aliasing starts proximal to the valve and the narrow band is directed from the orifice.*

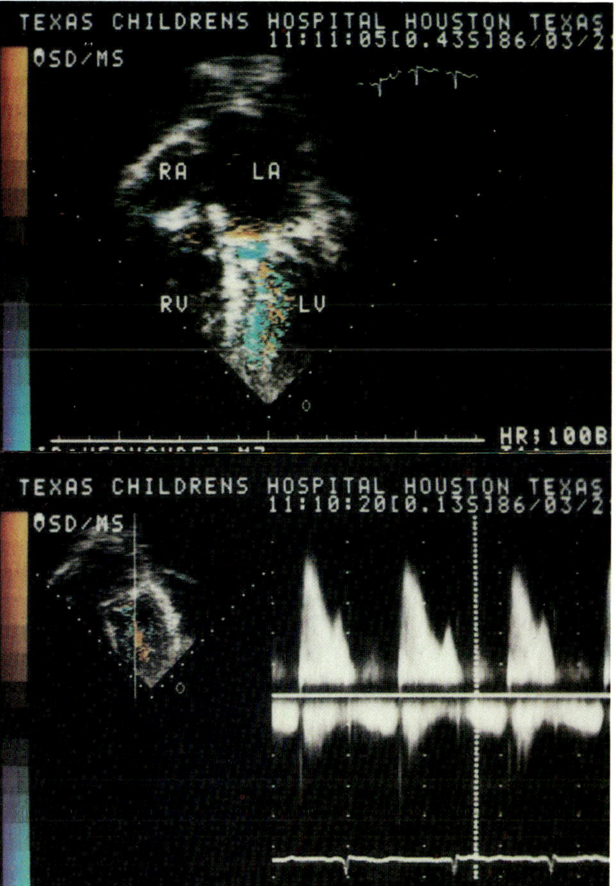

FIGURE 3-20—*Apical four-chamber view of a patient with mild mitral stenosis following repair of a large ventricular septal defect. Note the aliasing phenomenon that occurs proximal to the valve in the jet in the left ventricle of more widened appearance. Directed continuous-wave Doppler aligned parallel to the jet confirms the diagnosis of mild mitral stenosis with a peak velocity of 2.2 meters per second. LA = left atrium; LV = left ventricle; RA = right atrium; RV = right ventricle.*

orifice mitral valve,[14] and cor triatriatum. Both mitral stenosis and aortic regurgitation produce a high-velocity jet into the left ventricle in diastole but this jet can be differentiated easily when using color Doppler by gating in multiple phases of diastole.

In conclusion, color Doppler is helpful in mitral stenosis for the characterization of the flow, its direction, velocity, and turbulence. Directed continuous-wave Doppler using the jet as the guideline for alignment provides an accurate evaluation of the pressure gradient and mitral valve area.

Tricuspid Valve Stenosis

The presence of tricuspid valve stenosis is nonin-

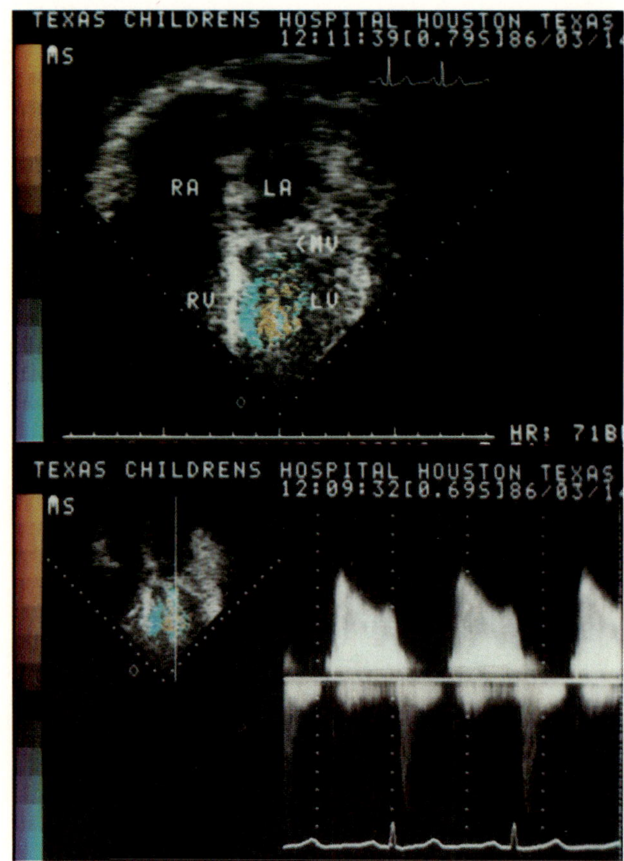

FIGURE 3-21—*Apical four-chamber view of a 15-year- old with rheumatic mitral stenosis. The variance mode with the typical flame or candle-like appearance of the jet during diastole is present. Note the mushroom appearance of the jet compared with the narrow band jet in the candle flame appearance (Figure 3-22). Continuous-wave Doppler confirms significant mitral stenosis and trivial mitral regurgitation. LA = left atrium; LV = left ventricle; MV = mitral valve; RA = right atrium; RV = right ventricle.*

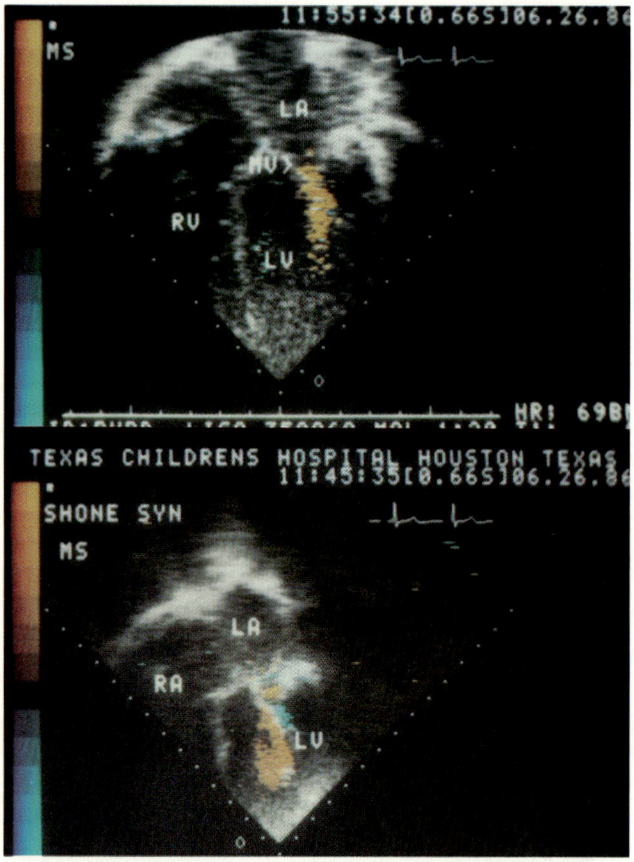

FIGURE 3-22—*Left ventricular inflow obstruction from a supra-mitral ring in association with aortic stenosis (Shone's syndrome). Gated diastolic frames show the "flame" appearance of mitral stenosis.*

vasively diagnosed using two-dimensional Doppler echocardiography. The apical four-chamber view is the preferable window for evaluation of this lesion and is supplemented by subcostal and parasternal projections. During the Doppler examination, velocities as high as in mitral stenosis are usually not found, but the Doppler display is clearly different from the normal tricuspid flow with two components. The rapid early filling and atrial systole have different color displays when the atrial kick is of high velocity (Figure 3-23).

From the maximum Doppler velocity recorded, the pressure may be calculated as in other obstructions using the modified Bernoulli equation but the compliance of the systemic circulation makes pressure gradient alone an inadequate parameter. Some estimate of cardiac output is needed in assessing this lesion.

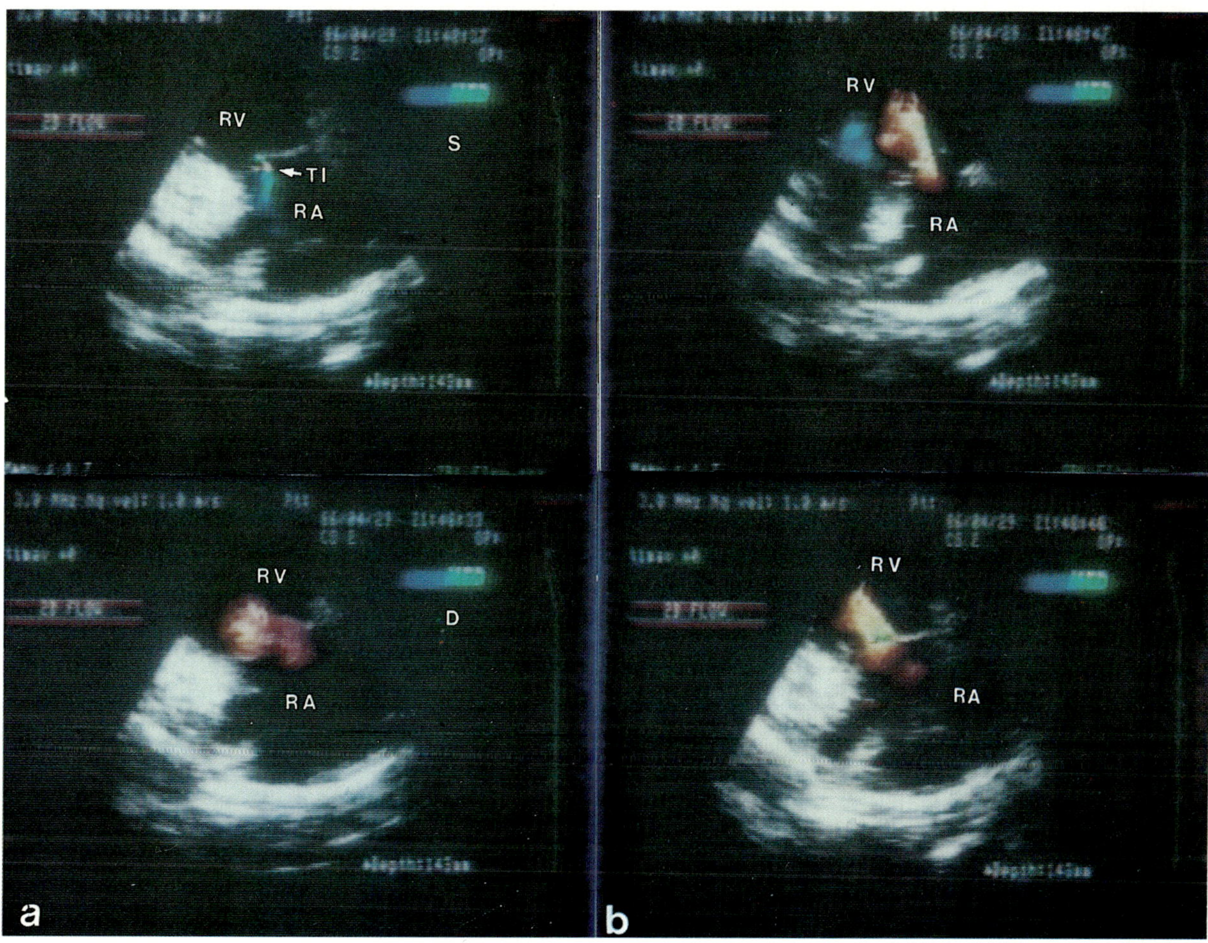

FIGURE 3-23—*Tricuspid valve stenosis (a) A systolic (S) frame shows trivial tricuspid regurgitation at the tricuspid valve (upper panel). Early diastolic filling of the right ventricle (RV) from the right atrium (RA) is seen in early diastole (D) (lower panel). (b) Early diastole (D) (upper panel) and late diastole (D) (lower panel) with tricuspid stenosis. Note the narrow high-velocity (yellow color) jet during atrial systole (S) (lower panel). (Reproduced by courtesy of Arthur E. Weyman, M.D., Massachusetts General Hospital, Boston, MA.)*

References

1. Hatle L, Angelsen B: Doppler Ultrasound in Cardiology—Physical Principles and Clinical Applications, 2nd ed. Philadelphia, Lea & Febiger, 1985.
2. Holen J, Simonsen S: Determination of pressure gradient in mitral stenosis with Doppler echocardiography. Br Heart J 41:529, 1979.
3. Teirstein P, Yock PG, Popp RL: The accuracy of Doppler ultrasound measurement of pressure gradients across irregular, dual and tunnel-like obstructions to blood flow. Circulation 72:577-584, 1985.
4. Segal J, Lerner DJ, Alderman El, et al: When is Doppler-determined valve area better than the Gorlin formula? Circulation 72(4):III-145, 1985(abstr).
5. Segal J, Lerner D, Miller DC, et al: Quantitation of hydraulic constants in the Gorlin and Holen-Hatle equations is important in low output states. Circulation 72(4):III-373, 1985 (abstr).
6. Young JB, Quinones MA, Waggoner AD, et al: Diagnosis and quantification of aortic stenosis with pulsed Doppler echocardiography. Am J Cardiol 45:987-994, 1980.
7. Vevrat C, Cholot N, Abitbol G, Kalmanson D: Non-invasive diagnosis and assessment of aortic valve disease and evaluation of aortic prosthesis function using echo pulsed Doppler velocimetry. Br Heart J 43:393-413, 1980.
8. Stevenson JG, Kawabori I: Noninvasive determination of pressure gradients in children: Two methods employing pulsed Doppler echocardiography. J Am Coll Cardiol 3:179-192, 1984.
9. Miyatake K, Okamoto M, Kinoshita N, et al: Clinical applications of a new type of real-time two-dimensional Doppler flow imaging system. Am J Cardiol 54:857-868, 1984.

10. Lima CO, Sahn DJ, Valdes-Cruz LM, et al: Noninvasive prediction of transvalvular pressure gradient in patients with pulmonary stenosis by quantitative two-dimensional echocardiographic Doppler studies. Circulation 67:866-871, 1983.
11. Richards KL, Scott RC, Crawford MH, et al: Non-invasive diagnosis of aortic and mitral valve disease with pulsed Doppler spectral analysis. Am J Cardiol 51:1122, 1983.
12. Richards KL, Cannon SR, Crawford MH, et al: Non-invasive diagnosis of aortic and mitral valve disease with pulsed Doppler spectral analysis. Am J Cardiol 51:1122-1127, 1983.
13. Khandheria BK, Tajik AJ, Reeder GS, et al: Doppler color flow imaging: A new technique for visualization and characterization of the blood flow jet in mitral stenosis. Mayo Clin Proc 61:623-630, 1986.
14. Reeder GS, Currie PJ, Hager DJ, et al: Use of Doppler techniques (continuous-wave pulsed-wave, and color flow imaging) in the noninvasive hemodynamic assessment of congenital heart disease. Mayo Clin Proc 61:725-744, 1986.

Chapter 4

Valvular Regurgitation

Robert Morrow, M.D.

There is no more potentially useful application of color-encoded Doppler flow mapping than the detection and quantification of valvular regurgitation. Conventional pulsed and continuous-wave Doppler have proven to be very sensitive and specific methods of detecting both atrioventricular and semilunar valve regurgitation.[1] In addition to detection of abnormal velocity patterns, semiquantitation of regurgitation with pulsed and continuous-wave Doppler allows estimation of volume flow and pressure gradients. However, conventional Doppler methods suffer from several important limitations. First, detection and quantification of valve regurgitation by conventional pulsed Doppler involves a meticulous process of searching the area of interest with the Doppler sample volume from different echocardiographic views. Since regurgitation jets are often eccentric and vary in shape, a cursory examination could lead to a false-negative diagnosis.[2] A complete examination, therefore, becomes time-consuming and tedious, especially when all four valves are examined. With continuous-wave Doppler, the lack of range resolution leads to a superimposition of regurgitation on other patterns of flow velocity which the ultrasound beam transects. Second, conventional pulsed Doppler, with or without range resolution, samples along a single axis and therefore provides information in essentially only one dimension.

Color-encoded multigate Doppler offers several potential advantages over conventional Doppler in the assessment of valvular regurgitation. Color Doppler allows simultaneous visualization of velocity data from multiple "sample volumes" along many axes. This allows representation of events during the cardiac cycle in two dimensions. The simultaneous representation of these events in real time obviates the need for meticulously mapping the area of interest with a single sample volume. This is a potentially time-saving procedure, particularly when all four cardiac valves must be examined. In addition, the two-dimensional representation of velocity, and hence flow, permits the development of a map of the regurgitant jet within the cardiac chamber without having to trace it by varying sample volume position.

The color method, however, is also not without limitations. Color Doppler is subject to all the depth and angle considerations that limit the use of conventional Doppler. In addition, the actual quantitation of velocity by color coding using the autocorrelation method is inferior to spectral analysis. Color Doppler does preserve the directional information provided by the Doppler signal. However, because of the low pulse repetition rate used in this format, frequency aliasing occurs at lower frequency shifts, and therefore at lower velocities, than with conventional Doppler.[3] When this occurs, as with conventional pulsed Doppler, the color coding of direction becomes ambiguous. In the majority of regurgitant lesions, high velocities lead to frequency aliasing which produces jets with ambiguous color coding. These are usually represented as alternating rings of red and blue regardless of the direction of the jet. Since most of these regurgitant jets are also turbulent, the mosaic pattern is frequently seen when the variance mode is used. Additional confusion may result from the fact that color change (aliasing) will occur based entirely on the depth of the interrogation. The jet of mitral regurgitation, for example, is of high velocity from the valve to the furthest extent of the jet in the left atrium. If the depth of sampling is increasing, as in a four-chamber projection, then jet mapping will be different at the greatest depth without a change in velocity.

When viewed in real time, color Doppler displays a large amount of complex information occurring during the cardiac cycle. This is particularly true in patients with rapid heart rates. For the unaccustomed observer, this can be very confusing. Gating during the cardiac cycle is helpful in studying these complex events but may be misleading. For example, a jet of regurgitation that occurs only during mid-systole may be overlooked if the image is gated only in early systole.

Nonetheless, initial experience with color Doppler suggests that it will be useful in both detection and quantification of regurgitation, even when used only with a velocity map with variance. In this chapter we summarize our experience and that of others with the use of color Doppler in patients with valvular regurgitation.

We specifically illustrate the use of color Doppler in pediatric patients with congenital heart disease. With each lesion we describe the optimal echocardiographic views for demonstrating regurgitation, with particular attention to depth and angle considerations. We also describe the appearance of the jet and the timing of regurgitation during the cardiac cycle. In addition, experience with quantitation of the severity of regurgitation using color Doppler is summarized.

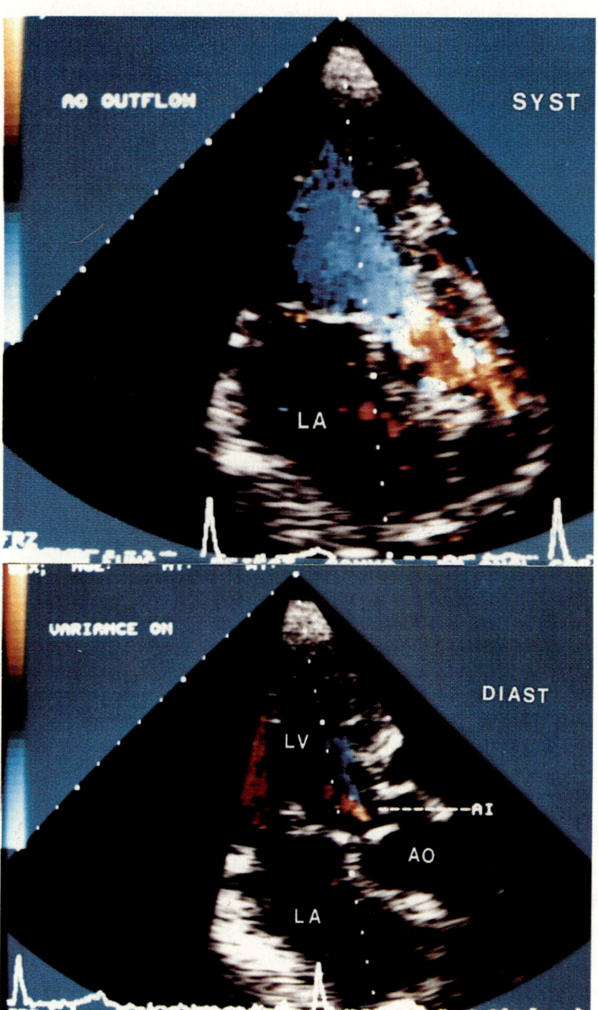

FIGURE 4-1—*Systole (upper) and diastole (lower) in a patient with aortic regurgitation. An apical four-chamber view shows the aortic regurgitation jet extending from the aortic valve through the left ventricular outflow tract into the body of the left ventricle (upper panel). The jet is a mosaic due to turbulence and frequency aliasing. In a long-axis view the regurgitation jet is seen extending along the anterior interventricular septum from the left ventricular outflow tract (lower panel). AO = aorta; AI = aortic insufficiency; LV = left ventricle; LA = left atrium; SYST = systole; DIAST = diastole.*

Aortic Regurgitation

The diastolic jet of aortic regurgitation may be detected from a variety of echocardiographic views, although no single view is ideal. The apical four-chamber view (Figure 4-1, upper panel) allows the smallest angle between the ultrasound beam and the jet of regurgitation but puts the aortic valve and left ventricular outflow tract at a significant distance from the transducer. This may lead to a loss of signal amplitude and an underrepresentation of the size of the jet. This is often a problem when examining large patients or patients with very large hearts and mild regurgitation. In contrast, the long-axis parasternal view (Figure 4-1, lower panel) allows detection of aortic regurgitation at the least depth but at the most unfavorable angle. However, visualization of regurgitation is possible from these views largely because of closer proximity of the transducer and the presence of turbulence in aortic regurgitation. A modified long-axis view from the low left parasternal position may reduce the angle between the ultrasound beam and the jet and thus allow better visualization of the jet than in the standard long-axis view, while maintaining the advantage of proximity between the area of interest and the transducer. Quantitation of the severity of aortic regurgitation is possible (see below) by comparing the size of the jet at the valve with the aortic annulus size as a ratio. As with angiography, the small, thin jet will be present when the amount of regurgitation is small (Figure 4-2) and a valve leak that is not localized is more severe (Figure 4-1). Even normal mitral valve diastolic filling of the left ventricle can mix with the aortic regurgitation jet, making it more difficult to quantitate.

Actual visualization of aortic regurgitation is usually not possible in adults from the suprasternal notch owing to the great depth of the left ventricular outflow tract from this transducer position, but in children with significant regurgitation this may be possible. Flow reversal in the ascending and descending aorta may be seen from the suprasternal notch, particularly in severe aortic regurgitation. It is important to remember that flow reversal may be seen in many lesions other than aortic regurgitation such as patent ductus arteriosus, cerebral arteriovenous malformations, aortopulmonary window, and surgically created systemic-to-pulmonary shunts (see Chapter 8).

Aortic regurgitation occurs in diastole after closure of the aortic leaflets. The principal determinants of the volume of the regurgitant fraction are the size of the defect in the closed aortic valve, the diastolic pressure gradient, and the length of the diastolic period. The velocity of the jet is determined, therefore, by the pressure gradient across the aortic valve in diastole. This

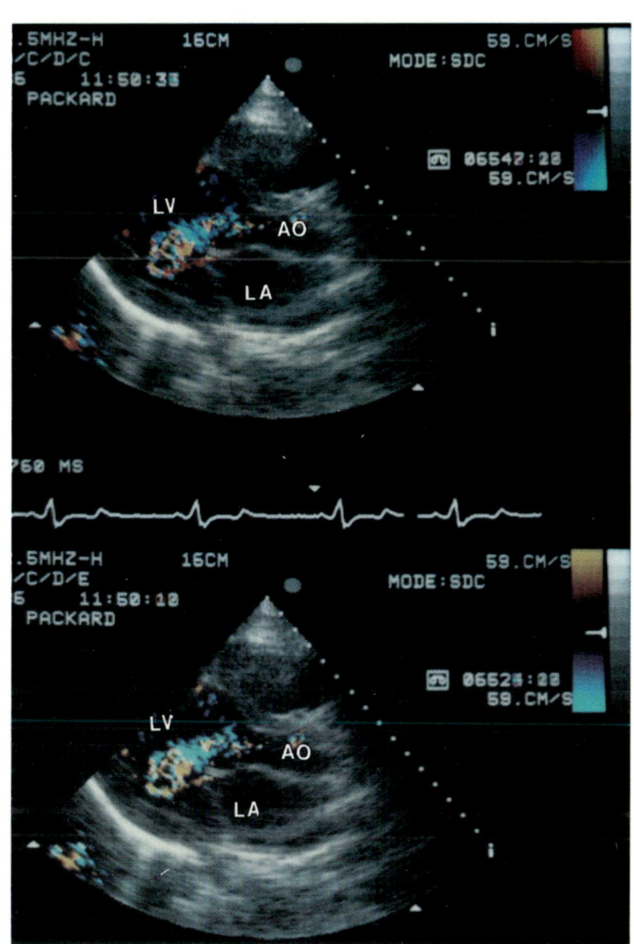

FIGURE 4-2—*Parasternal long-axis showing flow reversal in the left ventricular outflow tract in a patient with mild aortic regurgitation. Note the small site of origin of the jet at the aortic valve suggesting mild insufficiency. The color display without variance is shown for comparison (lower panel). AO = aorta; LA = left atrium; LV = left ventricle.*

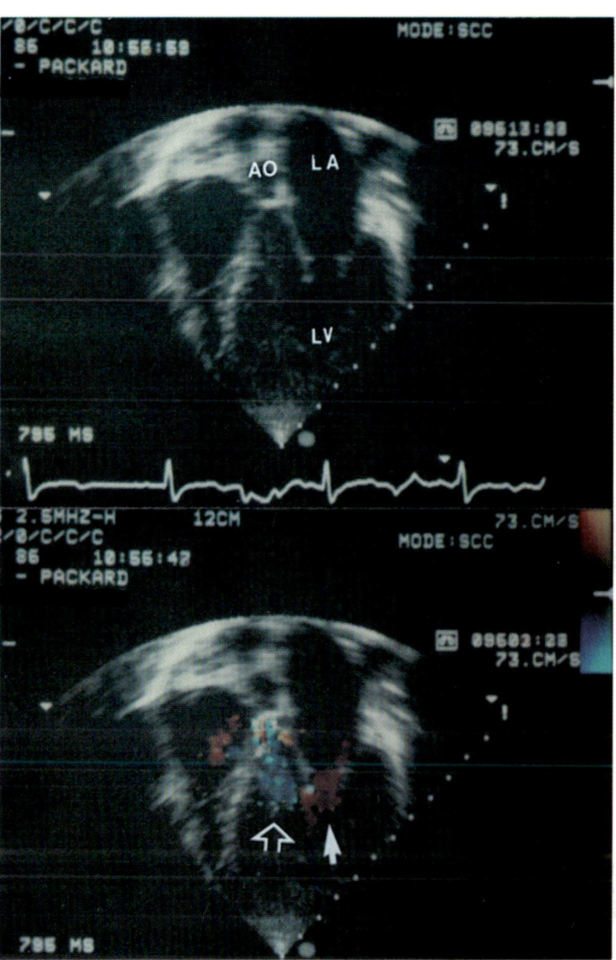

FIGURE 4-3—*A jet of aortic regurgitation viewed from the apex. The presence of a mosaic pattern in the left ventricular outflow tract is characteristic of aortic regurgitation (open white arrow). Two separate jets can be easily distinguished in the left ventricle using color Doppler; however, accurate measurement of the area of the aortic regurgitation jet can be difficult when mitral inflow mixes with it (white arrow). AO = aorta; LV = left ventricle; LA = left atrium.*

produces a turbulent, high-velocity jet which appears as a mosaic in the left ventricular outflow tract originating at the aortic valve and extending variable depths into the body of the left ventricle. The jet is most commonly directed through the center of the left ventricular outflow tract or along the ventricular septum (Figure 4-3). Occasionally, regurgitation may be directed toward the anterior leaflet of the mitral valve. This may result in confusion with either normal mitral valve inflow during diastole or with the jet of mitral stenosis. However, mitral valve inflow and the jet of mitral stenosis are usually directed from the mitral annulus to the apex. Consequently, it is usually possible to distinguish the jet of aortic regurgitation from mitral stenosis, and coexisting mitral stenosis and aortic regurgitation are uncommon in the pediatric age group.

In adults, aortic regurgitation most commonly occurs as a result of chronic rheumatic heart disease, following surgery for calcific aortic stenosis, or as a sequela of aortic valve endocarditis. The spectrum of aortic valve regurgitation, however, is somewhat different in pediatric patients. Rheumatic valvular disease is extremely uncommon in pediatric patients. Aortic regurgitation in this age group is usually the result of surgical valvotomy for congenital aortic stenosis (Figure 4-3). However, aortic regurgitation following aortic valve endocarditis does occur in this age group (Figure 4-4). Aortic regurgitation may also occur in patients with ventricular septal defects

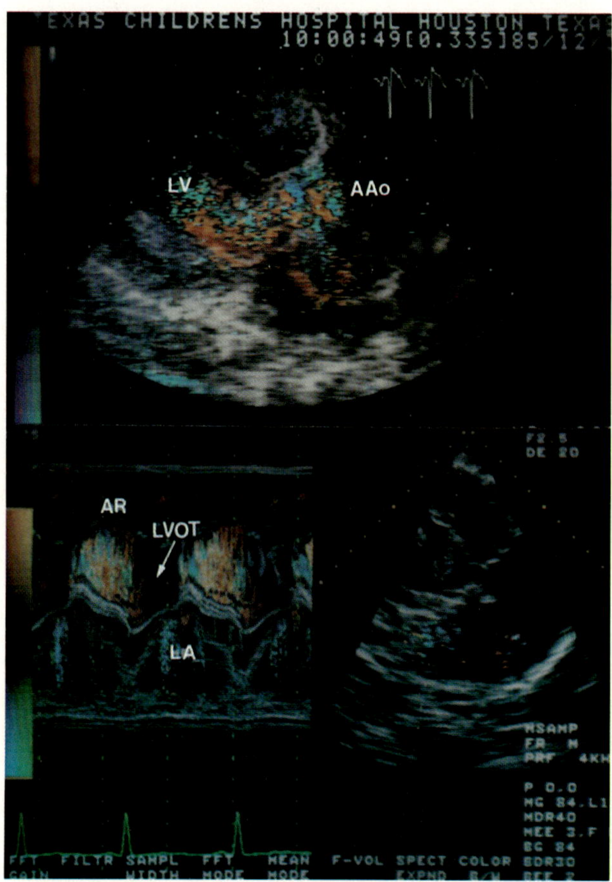

FIGURE 4-4—*Color Doppler images from the apex in a patient following treatment for aortic valve endocarditis. A broad jet can be seen extending well into the left ventricle, implying that at least a moderate degree of regurgitation is present. Color M-mode shows the variance findings in the left ventricular outflow tract (lower panel). AAO = ascending aorta; LV = left ventricle; LA = left atrium.*

in whom regurgitation is due to prolapse of the right aortic valve cusp. It is usually difficult to predict which patients with ventricular septal defects will develop aortic regurgitation, although the occurrence of aortic regurgitation is more commonly associated with supracristal ventricular septal defects. Color Doppler flow mapping may be particularly useful for the early detection of regurgitation in this setting. The other group of patients with systemic valve regurgitation have truncus arteriosus and truncal valve regurgitation (see Chapter 6).

Estimates of the *severity* of aortic regurgitation using pulsed Doppler to map the depth of extension of the regurgitation jet into the left ventricle have been shown to correlate well with angiographic grading of severity.[1,4,5] Pulsed Doppler mapping of regurgitation involves moving the sample volume from the aortic annulus through the left ventricle outflow tract to the body of the ventricular cavity. Grading systems are based on the depth of penetration of the jet into the left ventricle. The process of mapping regurgitation with pulsed Doppler is tedious and time-consuming. In addition, the diastolic flow disturbance may be contaminated with mitral inflow or with the jet of mitral stenosis leading to ambiguity. The regurgitant fraction in aortic regurgitation can also be estimated by the ratio of forward to reverse flow on pulsed Doppler examination of the ascending or descending aorta.[6-9] However, this method is useful primarily for distinguishing mild from severe regurgitation and is confined to pure aortic regurgitation when Doppler interrogation is performed in the ascending aorta.[6]

Color Doppler has been shown to be both sensitive and specific for aortic regurgitation, with sensitivity ranging from 75 to 100 percent.[10-14] In addition, a number of investigators have evaluated the use of color Doppler in the estimation of the severity of aortic regurgitation by comparing color Doppler to angiographic quantitation. Much of this information has been collected in adults and represents preliminary work. It appears, however, that there is a relationship between severity of regurgitation as assessed by these two methods. Omoto found an excellent correlation between angiography and depth of extension of the regurgitation jet into the body of the left ventricle.[13] Others have evaluated the width and area of the regurgitation jet in an attempt to predict severity. Byard et al.[15] found a good correlation between the ratio of width of the regurgitation jet to width of the left ventricular outflow tract and angiographic grading of severity in 21 adult patients with aortic regurgitation (Figure 4-4). These investigators also found a poor correlation between length and long-axis area and angiographic grading. In a similar study, Perry et al.[16] found a strong correlation between the ratio of area of the regurgitation jet to left ventricular outflow tract area in the short axis compared to angiography. Pearlman et al.[17] also found a relationship between jet width and severity. In their study, patients with significant aortic regurgitation never had narrow jets although some with mild aortic regurgitation had moderate or broad jets. Yock[10] found it difficult to measure the area of the regurgitation jet because of contamination by mitral inflow. In a different approach, Brouchard[18] calculated regurgitant volume from the color flow map of aortic regurgitation using Simpson's rule. Regurgitant volume by color Doppler was compared to blood pool scintigraphy. In this study the two methods correlated closely ($r = 0.88$). Mild regurgitation jet is confined to the region immediately subadjacent to the aortic valve, whereas the severe regurgitation jet is wide, extends along the ventricular septum, and penetrates deep into the body of the left ventricle. Moderate regurgitation is intermediate in width and depth.

In general, it appears that the size of the regurgitation jet compares favorably with invasive estimates of regurgitant fraction. However, the ability to predict severity has not been conclusively demonstrated. This may in part be because angiographic grading in itself is semiquantitative and subjective, but may also be because the color Doppler method is based on a velocity map that does not reflect the quantity of regurgitation directly. Also, changes in afterload and heart rate between the time of the echocardiographic examination and the time of catheterization could profoundly affect the degree of aortic regurgitation. In addition, clinical severity of aortic regurgitation is often related to coexisting lesions and underlying impairment of myocardial function and not strictly proportional to regurgitant fraction. For example, after aortic valvotomy the continued presence of significant stenosis can affect the myocardial function. Continuous-wave Doppler can quantitate the gradient from the left ventricle to the aorta but some allowance for the increased volume of ejection due to the aortic regurgitation is necessary (Figure 4-5). Further work in this large group of pediatric patients is necessary. The contribution of color Doppler to the serial evaluation of aortic regurgitation in individual patients and the effect of this modality on patient selection for valve replacement remains to be determined. Future work should emphasize the use of Doppler displays that map the intensity of the Doppler signal to better represent the volume of regurgitant flow.

In summary, visualization of aortic regurgitation requires imaging in at least three echocardiographic views to assess the width and depth of the diastolic flow disturbance. By using a combination of views, the examiner can overcome the limitations of unfavorable depth of the aortic valve and left ventricular outflow tract and large angles between the ultrasound beam and the regurgitant jet.

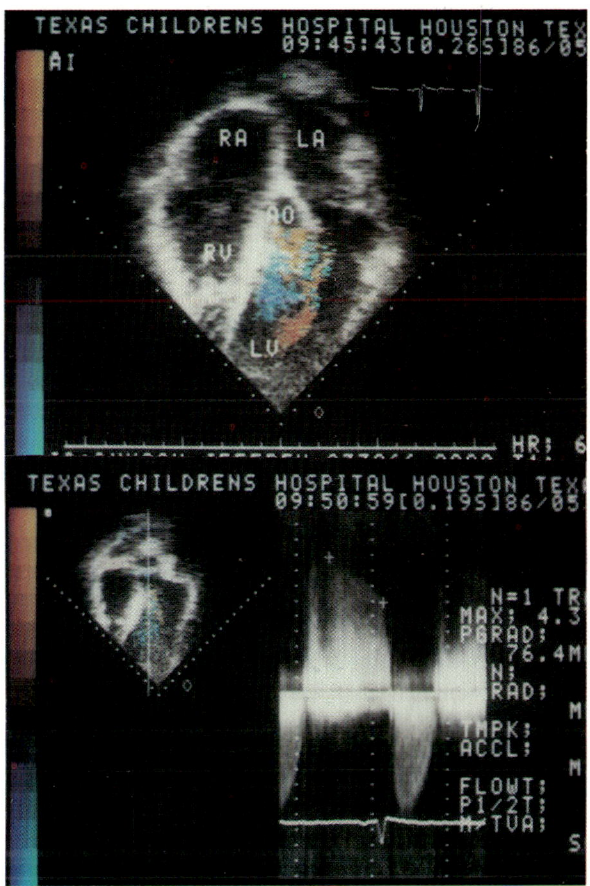

FIGURE 4-5—*Severe aortic regurgitation in the apical view. The left ventricular outflow tract is virtually filled with this mosaic jet. The jet is broad and extends deep into the body of the left ventricle. Continuous-wave Doppler aligned with the jet demonstrates the typical spectral display of aortic insufficiency. A systolic peak velocity of 4 meters per second is compatible with some degree of aortic stenosis as well. AV = aortic valve; LV = left ventricle; LA = left atrium.*

Pulmonary Regurgitation

Pulmonary regurgitation is visualized best from the parasternal short-axis view and from a modified parasternal long-axis view. Pulmonary regurgitation is readily seen in the short axis owing to the proximity of the transducer to the right ventricular outflow tract and the area immediately below the pulmonary valve. The modified long-axis view of the pulmonary artery is useful to demonstrate flow reversal in the pulmonary artery that occurs as a result of regurgitation. The use of higher-frequency transducers in pediatric patients (5 MHz) allows better focus in the near field and better signal-to-noise ratio. However, frequency aliasing occurs at lower velocities with higher-frequency transducers. Both views also allow a relatively favorable angle to flow. It is possible, particularly in small pediatric patients, to visualize the right ventricular outflow tract and the jet of pulmonary regurgitation from the subcostal view. Although this provides a minimal angle to flow, the right ventricular outflow tract is at considerable depth from the transducer. This frequently leads to low signal amplitude and poor imaging of the regurgitant jet, particularly in larger patients.

Pulmonary artery pressure, the size of the defect in the closed pulmonary valve, heart rate, and right ventricular compliance will all have an affect on the amount of regurgitation observed. In addition, variations in the degree of regurgitation will occur with respiration and may be altered in patients on positive pressure ventilation. Pulmonary regurgitation, like aortic regurgitation, occurs at closure of the semilunar valve leaflets. However, unlike aortic regurgitation, pulmonary regurgitation often occurs with a lower pressure gradient, particularly following valvotomy or valvectomy. As a result, the jet of pulmonary regurgitation is often lower in velocity and can be laminar. This is a useful method for estimating the diastolic pulmonary artery pressure by assuming the end-diastolic pressure in the right ventricle. When severe pulmonary regurgitation exists following valvotomy, holodiastolic regurgitation occurs with virtual equalization of pulmonary diastolic pressure and right ventricular end-diastolic pressure. With severe pulmonary hypertension, the high-velocity pulmonary regurgitation jet produces frequency aliasing and an ambiguous color display.

Mild pulmonary regurgitation in a normal patient is not uncommon and appears as a red jet directed toward the transducer in the parasternal short-axis view (Figure 4-6). However, a mosaic jet may be seen, particulary if pulmonary hypertension is present or if pulmonary regurgitation is severe, and this will determine whether the jet will be localized to the area just below the pulmonary valve or extend to a greater depth in the right ventricular outflow tract.

Pulmonary regurgitation is commonly observed in both adult and pediatric patients and can be demonstrated with both conventional and color Doppler in a large number of healthy subjects.[1,19,20] Using contrast enhancement of Doppler signals demonstrated that these findings were indeed related to right-sided regurgitation and were not due to coronary flow. In general, however, it appears that color Doppler may be less sensitive to small amounts of pulmonary regurgitation than pulsed Doppler.[10,21] In a majority of patients, mild pulmonary regurgitation is of no clinical significance.

Pulmonary regurgitation is frequently observed in congenital heart disease both in patients with pulmonary valvar disease and in patients with secondary pulmonary hypertension. The most commonly observed setting for significant pulmonary regurgitation is in patients who have undergone valvotomy for pulmonary stenosis or repair of tetralogy of Fallot (Figure 4-7). Following repair of tetralogy of Fallot, the degree of either distal or proximal residual pulmonary stenosis and the degree of secondary pulmonary regurgitation are of importance in assessing the operative repair. Under low pressure—that is, without distal obstruction—pulmonary regurgitation may appear as a homogeneous red jet. The presence of

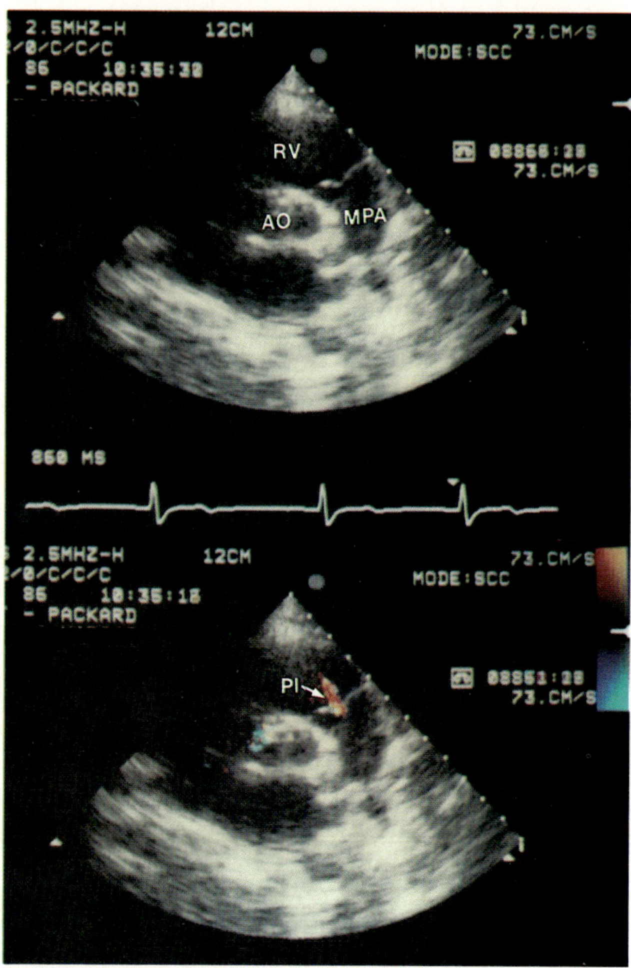

FIGURE 4-6—*Pulmonary regurgitation visualized from the parasternal short-axis view in a normal patient. This jet is a homogeneous red color well localized to the region just below the pulmonary valve. AO = aorta; MPA = main pulmonary artery; RV = right ventricle.*

a mosaic jet extending deep into the right ventricular outflow tract should lead to a further search for distal obstruction at the proximal pulmonary artery branches or in the lungs. A large mosaic jet of severe pulmonary regurgitation may be seen without significant distal obstruction if there is severe right ventricular dysfunction.

Pulmonary regurgitation is also observed in patients with either primary or secondary forms of pulmonary hypertension. The normal newborn has somewhat elevated pulmonary artery pressure and may have an aliased jet of pulmonary regurgitation (Figure 4-8). Patients with absent pulmonary valve syndrome have classic physical findings, usually permitting easy recognition of this unusual lesion on physical examination alone. Nonetheless, the color Doppler examination is

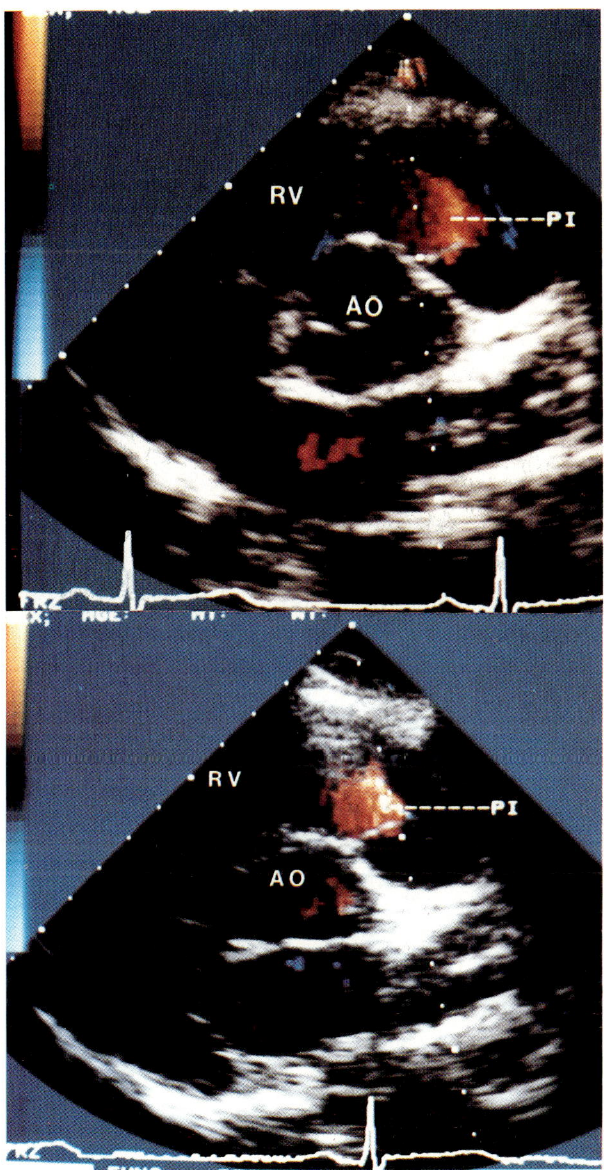

FIGURE 4-7—*Parasternal short-axis view with severe pulmonary regurgitation. A large mosaic jet is seen extending from the level of the pulmonary valve well into the right ventricular outflow tract (lower panel). AO = aorta; PI = pulmonary insufficiency; RV = right ventricle.*

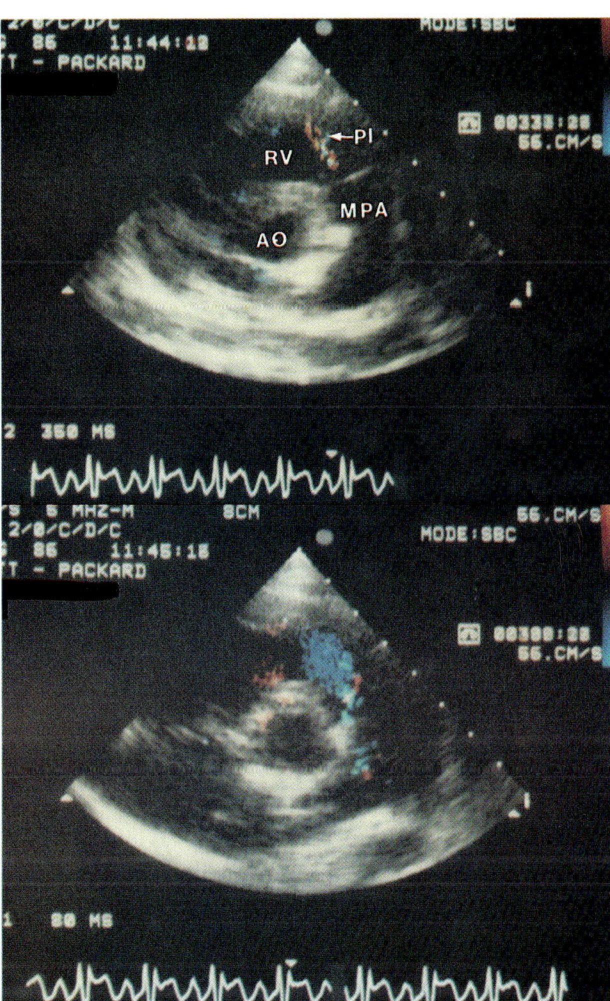

FIGURE 4-8—*Short-axis imaging of mild pulmonary regurgitation following repair for ventricular septal defect. A narrow red jet can be seen originating at the pulmonary valve and extending below the pulmonary valve (upper panel). In systole there is variance at the PV (lower panel). MPA = main pulmonary artery; RV = right ventricle; PI = pulmonary insufficiency.*

very striking because of the presence of both pulmonary stenosis and regurgitation (Figure 4-9).

Color Doppler, therefore, is useful in the detection of pulmonary regurgitation, although a significant number of normal individuals may have a visible diastolic flow disturbance in the right ventricular outflow tract. Clear criteria for grading the severity of pulmonary regurgitation are lacking. Takao[19] was successful in distinguishing pulmonary regurgitation due to pulmonary hypertension from pulmonary regurgitation in normal individuals by the extension of the jet into the right ventricular outflow tract. In this study of adults, the hypertensive pulmonary regurgitation jet extended more than two centimeters into the right ventricular outflow tract. It is likely that the width as well as the area of the regurgitation jet will prove to be useful in assessing severity. Although mild pulmonary regurgitation may be detected in normal individuals, the presence of a mosaic jet extending deep into the right ventricular outflow tract in patients without pulmonary valve disease should prompt a search for significant pulmonary hypertension.

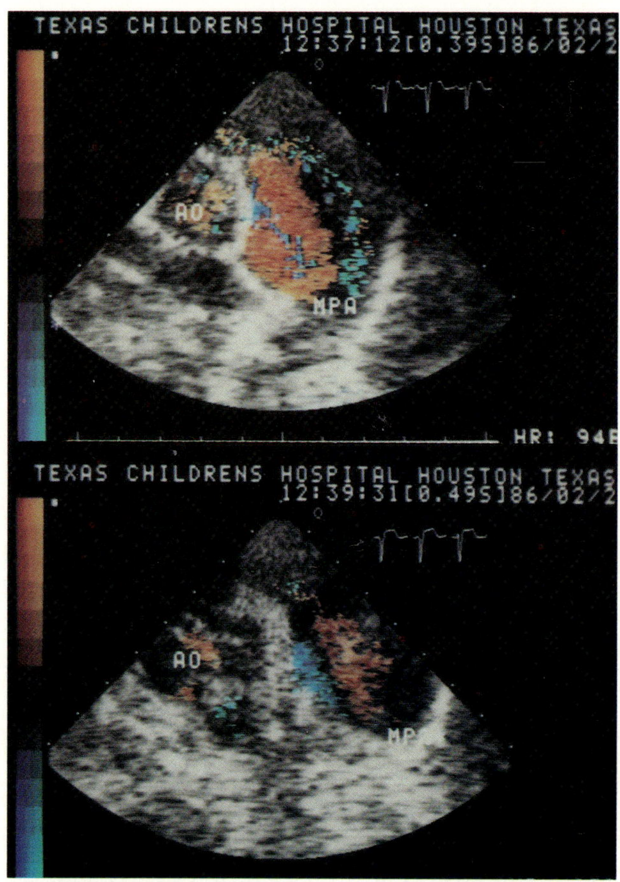

FIGURE 4-9—*Absent pulmonary valve syndrome produces both pumonary obstruction, due to dysplasia of the pulmonary valve or pulmonary annular hypoplasia, and pulmonary regurgitation. Systolic frames demonstrate turbulence and aliasing in the main pulmonary artery secondary to obstruction (upper panel). Diastolic frames show flow reversal in the pulmonary artery and a pulmonary regurgitation jet extending into the right ventricular outflow tract. Severe dilatation of the main pulmonary artery can be seen. AO = aorta; MPA = main pulmonary artery.*

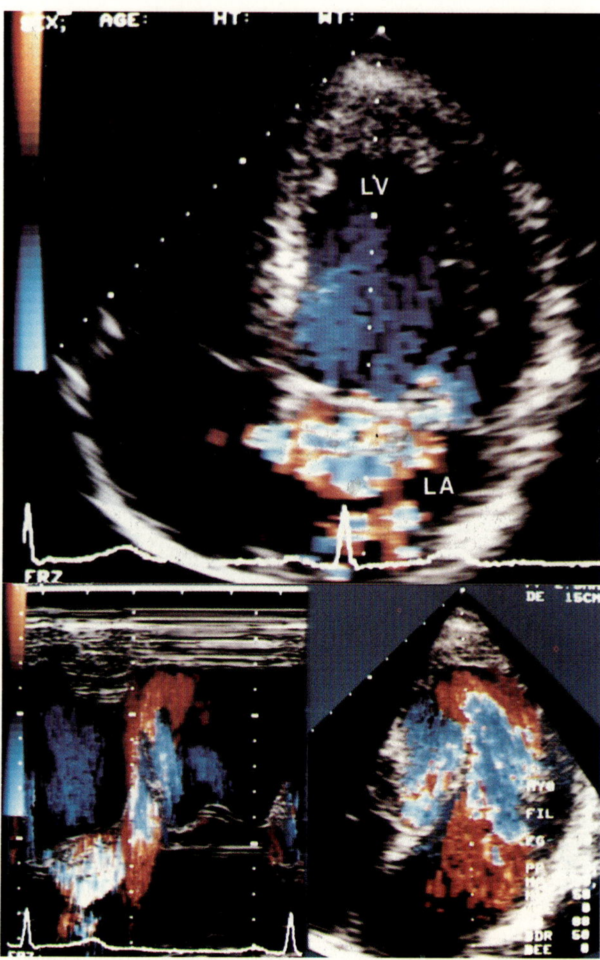

FIGURE 4-10—*Apical four-chamber view demonstrating mitral regurgitation. The jet appears as a mosaic originating and extending into the left atrium during systole (upper panel). Normal diastolic filling of the left ventricle is present (lower panel) with color M mode. LA = left atrium; LV = left ventricle.*

Mitral Regurgitation

Optimal visualization of the jet of mitral regurgitation may be obtained by a combination of apical and parasternal views. In most patients the jet of mitral regurgitation is directed from the apex to base. Thus, the apical view often gives the best angle to the axis of blood flow from left ventricle to left atrium (Figure 4-10). However, in some commonly encountered lesions such as mitral valve prolapse and complete or incomplete atrioventricular canal defects, the jet of mitral regurgitation may be eccentric. For example, mitral regurgitation secondary to mitral valve prolapse may be directed either anteriorly or posteriorly.[2] In patients with eccentric jets, the parasternal long-axis view may provide better visualization of the regurgitant jet (Figure 4-11). In both complete and incomplete atrioventricular canal defects mitral regurgitation is commonly observed and is due either to insufficient mitral valve tissue or to inadequate coaptation of valve leaflets. In this lesion the regurgitant jet is often directed either toward the atrial septum or to the right of the atrial septum (Figure 4-12). In patients with anteriorly directed eccentric jets, the parasternal long-axis view may provide better visualization. The parasternal long-axis view also places the transducer in closest proximity to the left atrium. Thus, this view is useful when poor color Doppler images are obtained from the apical view as a result of low signal amplitude. This may occur in older patients, in small patients with severe cardiomegaly, or in patients with prosthetic mitral valves and perivalvular leaks. However, except in patients with eccentric jets, the long-axis parasternal view offers a poor angle to regurgitant flow. A transducer position lower on the left parasternal border may improve the angle between the ultrasound beam and the jet. In patients with congenital heart defects with mitral regurgitation, all views should be tried because of the unpredictability of the jet direction or timing. The use of multiple views, particularly the long-axis and the apical views, allows three-dimensional spatial reconstruction of the regurgitant jet from the two-dimensional flow images. This is most important in complex forms of congenital heart disease where the orientation of the systemic atrioventricular valve is unusual,

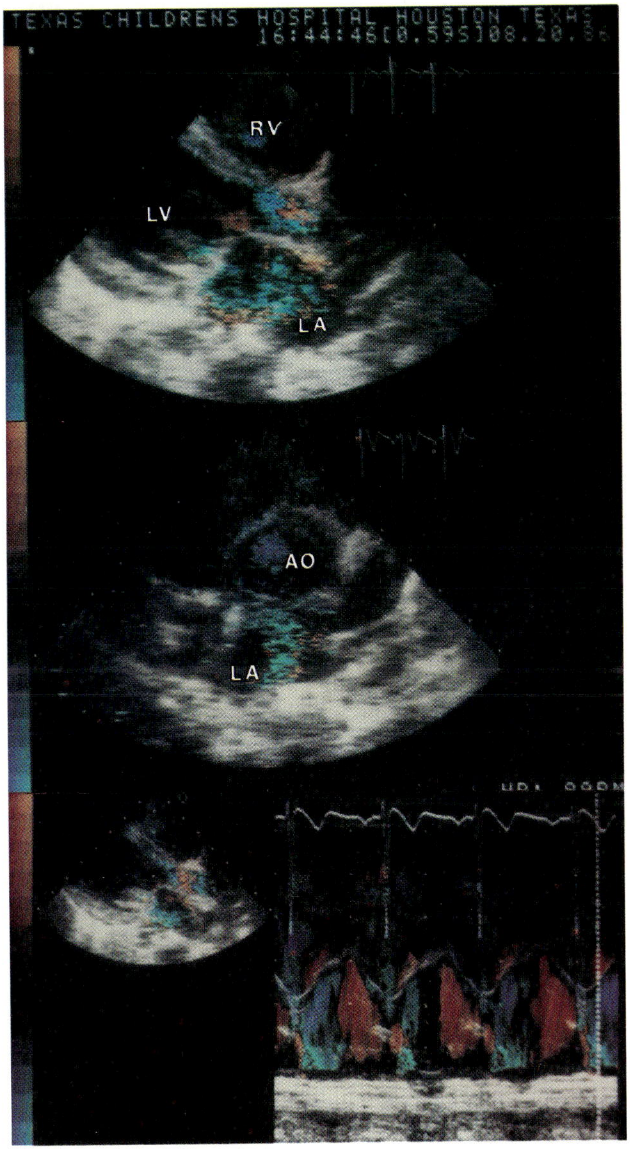

FIGURE 4-11—*Parasternal long-axis view demonstrating an eccentric mitral regurgitation jet in a patient with incomplete atrioventricular canal and a "cleft" mitral valve. The variance color (green) indicates that the jet is of high velocity and the direction is initially toward the left atrium and anterior deeper in the left atrium. Mitral regurgitation from the cleft mitral valve is seen also in a modified short-axis view (middle panel). Color M-mode confirms the holosystolic nature of the regurgitation (lower panel). LV = left ventricle; LA = left atrium; MV = mitral valve.*

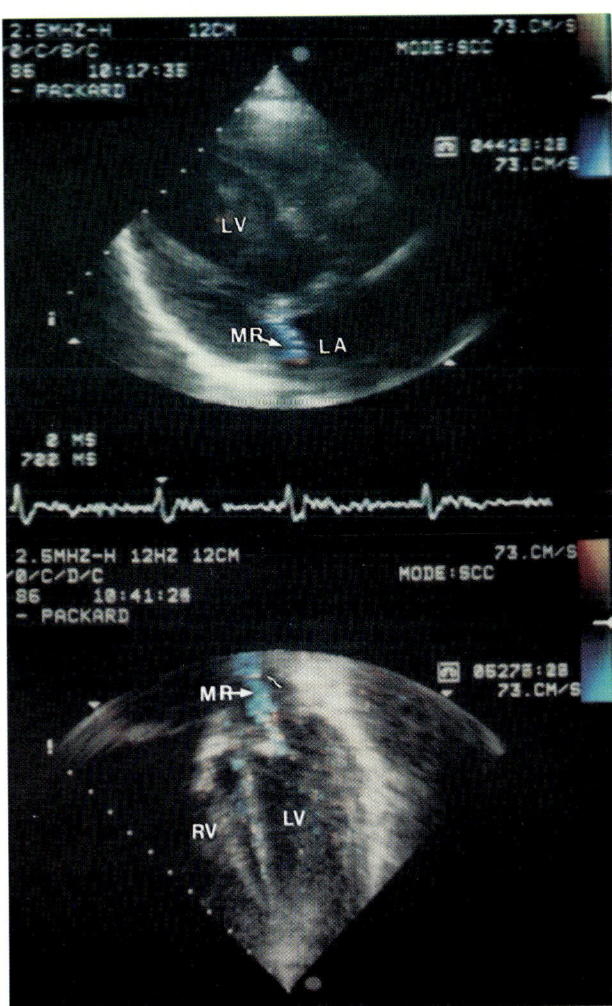

FIGURE 4-12—*Mild mitral regurgitation (MR) in a patient following repair of AV canal defect from the parasternal (upper panel) and apical four-chamber (lower panel) views. The image is gated in early systole. By combining views, the three-dimensional orientation of the jet can be estimated. Some jets change direction during systole and the timing of systolic gating should be scanned (see Figure 4-13). LV = left ventricle; LA = left atrium; MV = mitral valve.*

makaing the direction of the regurgitation jet difficult to predict (corrected transposition, dextrocardia; see Chapter 6).

As noted above, color Doppler flow images obtained in real time may be confusing to examiners who are unaccustomed to viewing the complex events that are displayed during the cardiac cycle in the color Doppler format. This is particularly true in pediatric patients who often have higher heart rates. Images that are obtained by gating to the cardiac cycle are often less difficult to interpret. It is important, however, to appreciate the timing of regurgitation, particularly when interpreting color Doppler images obtained by gating to the cardiac cycle. Mitral regurgitation begins at the onset of systole with closure of the mitral valve and is usually holosystolic. It has been estimated that over 50 percent of the regurgitant volume is ejected into the left atrium before the aortic valve opens.[22] However, in mitral valve prolapse the timing of mitral regurgitation is variable and may occur predominantly in mid- or late systole. By gating only in early systole the examiner may fail to detect regurgitation or may underestimate the severity of regurgitation due to mitral prolapse. Therefore, when real-time images are unclear and gating is used, it is important to gate throughout systole to adequately exclude mitral regurgitation (Figure 4-13). Thus, the method of gating could significantly alter the planimeterized area obtained when estimating severity of regurgitation. Even in the presence of moderate or severe elevation of left atrial pressure, the jet of mitral regurgitation is a high-velocity jet, reflecting systolic left ventricular pressure. The resultant frequency aliasing and turbulence produce a mosaic pattern in the variance mode regardless of the echocardiographic view. The jet is usually elliptical or circular and directed apex to base, although, as noted above, the regurgitant jet may be eccentric and take a variety of shapes.[2]

In the pediatric age group, isolated mitral regurgitation is a relatively uncommon lesion; mitral valve regurgitation, however, usually occurs in association with other congenital lesions such as coarctation of the aorta or complete or incomplete atrioventricular canal. Thus, in cases of complete atrioventricular canal, color Doppler may be useful in the preoperative evaluation in estimating the severity of mitral regurgitation, tricuspid regurgitation, and the left ventricular to right atrial shunt. Systemic atrioventricular valve regurgitation in patients with atrioventricular discordance (corrected transposition, ventricular inversion) is physiologically similar to mitral regurgitation, even though there is abnormal valve morphology (usually tricuspid or "Ebstein-like"; see Chapter 6). Mitral regurgitation may be present in infants with anomalous left coronary artery (Figures 4-16 and 4-17). Mitral regurgitation occurs in these patients as a result of papillary muscle infarction and ventricular dilatation (see Chapter 9). Although commonly observed in the pediatric and adolescent age groups, mitral valve prolapse rarely results in hemodynamically significant mitral regurgitation in the pediatric patient but can be acquired after rheumatic fever.

Conventional pulsed and continuous-wave Doppler have been shown to be highly sensitive and specific in the detection of mitral regurgitation.[1,7,23] Likewise, the majority of investigators have found color Doppler flow imaging to be both sensitive and specific for mitral regurgitation and to agree with findings on pulsed Doppler examination in individual patients.[10,13,14,24] However, reported sensitivity ranges from 67 to 94

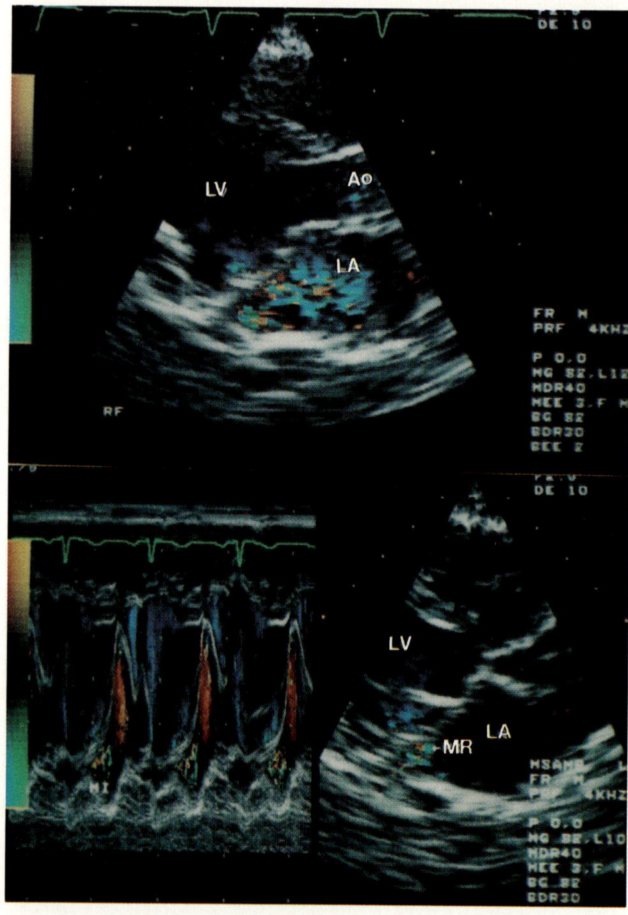

FIGURE 4-13—*Mitral regurgitation (MR) following acute rheumatic fever in a 12-year-old boy. The area of the left atrium filled by the velocity/variance jet varies depending on the projection (compare upper and lower panels) and the timing in systole. The latter is well defined for any given line by color M-mode (left lower panel). Ao = aorta; LA = left atrium; LV = left ventricle.*

percent and specificity ranges from 78 to 100 percent when compared to angiography.

Mitral regurgitation may be graded using pulsed Doppler by assessing the intensity of the Doppler spectral signal, analysis of the effect of regurgitation on the aortic velocity profile, and by mapping the jet of regurgitation in the left atrium.[1,23] Each of these methods is in effect a semiquantitative estimate of the regurgitant fraction. However, mapping of regurgitation with pulsed Doppler is a tedious and time-consuming process. Color flow Doppler mapping offers the potential advantage of visualizing the flow disturbance in the left atrium caused by mitral regurgitation in two dimensions rather than in one dimension. Recent studies have sought to correlate the size of the jet of mitral regurgitation with the size of the regurgitant fraction by angiography.[10,14,25] These studies have been performed almost exclusively in adults with either rheumatic heart disease or mitral valve prolapse and it is not known if they may be directly applicable to congential defects. Saenz et al.[25] found that the planimeterized area of regurgitation correlated well with the regurgitant fraction estimated angiographically. By measuring area alone, the authors were able to separate mild from severe regurgitation but were unable to distinguish mild from moderate regurgitation. The averaged ratio of the area of the regurgitation jet to the area of the left atrium from at least two views provided a better differentiation of the three grades of mitral regurgitation.[14] However, these authors found a poor correlation between maximum length or width of the jet and the severity of regurgitation by angiography. In another study comparing maximum length, area, and the ratio of area of the jet to area of the left atrium to angiography, a poor correlation was found for all three methods.[10] Certainly, in a patient with isolated mitral disease, when the jet of tricuspid regurgitation by continuous-wave Doppler exceeds that of the mitral regurgitation (Figure 4-14), then the degree of mitral regurgitation is severe.

There are several possible explanations for these varying results. First, as in the case of aortic regurgitation, angiographic grading systems are usually subjective and are semiquantitative at best. Second, changes in afterload, myocardial function, and heart rate and rhythm could produce dynamic changes in regurgitation, resulting in differences between color Doppler mapping and angiographic grading. Low signal amplitude or a large angle between the ultrasound beam and the regurgitation may cause substantial underestimation of the area. Clearly, the best representation of the severity of regurgitation will be obtained when two or more views are combined with a careful examination of the size of the jet throughout systole. It is important to remember that in individual patients the regurgitant volume may not correlate with clinical severity. This is particularly true in congenital heart disease where multiple lesions may coexist. In addition, pediatric patients with congenital heart disease usually do not have underlying ischemic heart disease. Serial estimates of the severity of regurgitation by color Doppler may prove to be more useful clinically than an absolute quantitation of regurgitant volume.

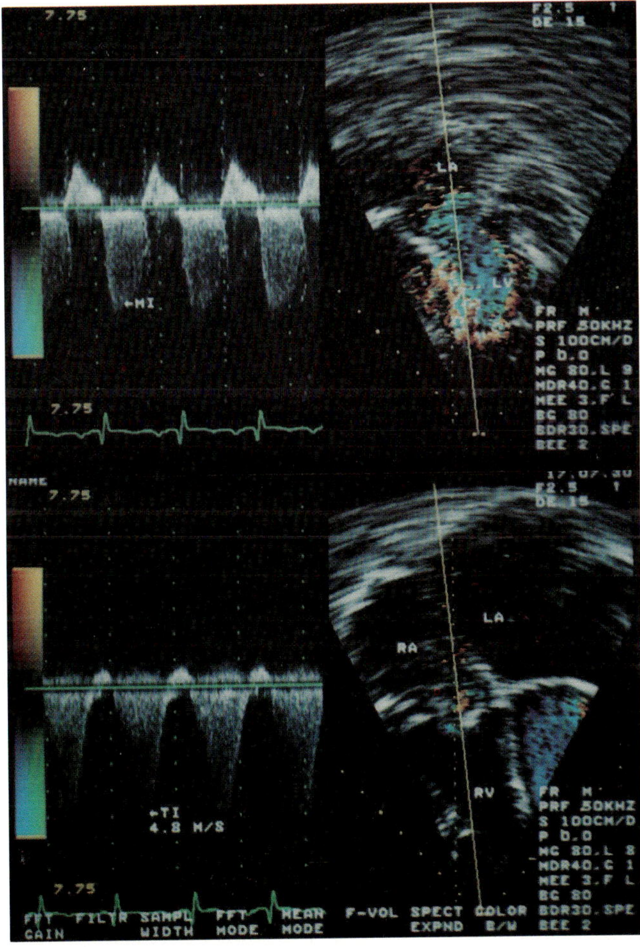

FIGURE 4-14—*Severe mitral regurgitation due to rheumatic fever using color Doppler-directed continous-wave Doppler. The mitral regurgitation (MR-upper panel with a diastolic frame) has a peak velocity of 4 meters per second while the jet of tricuspid regurgitation (TR; lower panel) has a velocity of 4.8 meters per second (higher) indicative of severe pulmonary hypertension. Note the increased diastolic filling velocities of the mitral tracing. LA = left atrium; LV = left ventricle; RA = right atrium; RV = right venticle.*

Tricuspid Regurgitation

The apical four-chamber and the parasternal short-axis views provide the best orientation to visualize the jet of tricuspid regurgitation. From the apical four-chamber view an excellent angle to flow can be obtained in the majority of cases (Figure 4-15). This view also allows clear differentiation of tricuspid from mitral regurgitation in patients with complete atrioventricular canal. However, as in the case of mitral regurgitation, the distance of the tricuspid valve from the transducer in the apical view may lead to loss of signal amplitude with currently available equipment. This is more likely to occur in patients with minimal amounts of tricuspid regurgitation and normal right ventricular pressure. The parasternal short-axis view may overcome some of this difficulty with depth. In addition, a good angle to flow is obtained with this view in the majority of cases. Subcostal imaging often complements the parasternal short-axis and apical views.

In the short-axis view the jet of tricuspid regurgitation is often close to the aortic root and represents regurgitation through the area of the septal leaflet of the tricuspid valve. In patients with right ventricular hypertension, the tricuspid regurgitation jet will have alternating rings of blue and red with varying intensity due to frequency aliasing (Figure 4-16). In these patients turbulence will lead to a mosaic pattern in the variance mode. Thus, it may be possible to exclude significant right ventricular hypertension if a homogeneous blue localized tricuspid regurgitation jet is observed.

It is important to distinguish tricuspid regurgitation from other sources of systolic flow in the right atrium.

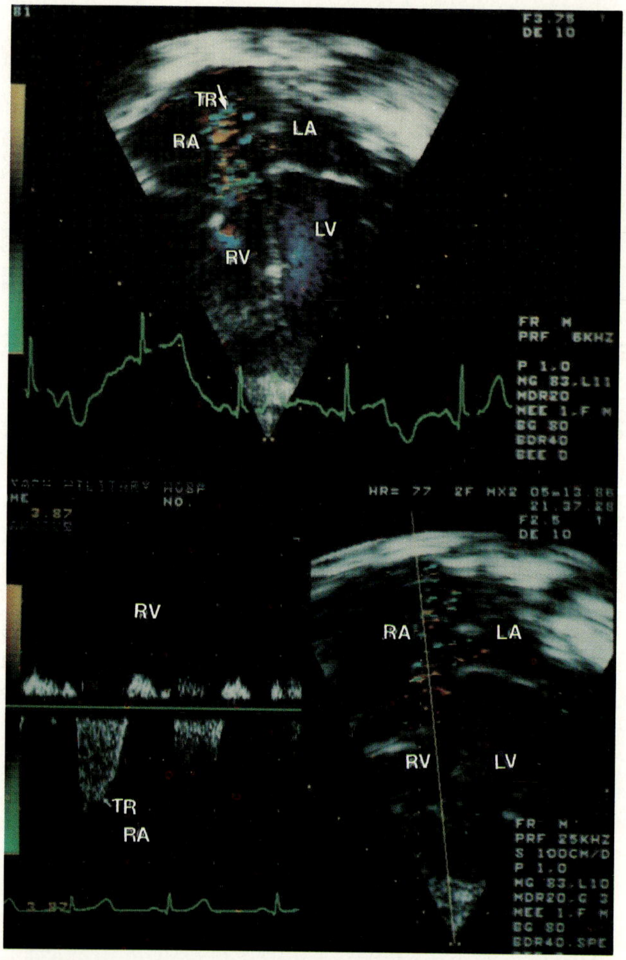

FIGURE 4-15—*Tricuspid regurgitation (TR) visualized from the apical four-chamber view. Variance in the jet is present (upper panel) and the peak velocity is low (2 meters per second), indicating the absence of increased right ventricular pressure. LA = left atrium; LV = left ventricle; RV = right ventricle; RA = right atrium; TV = tricuspid valve.*

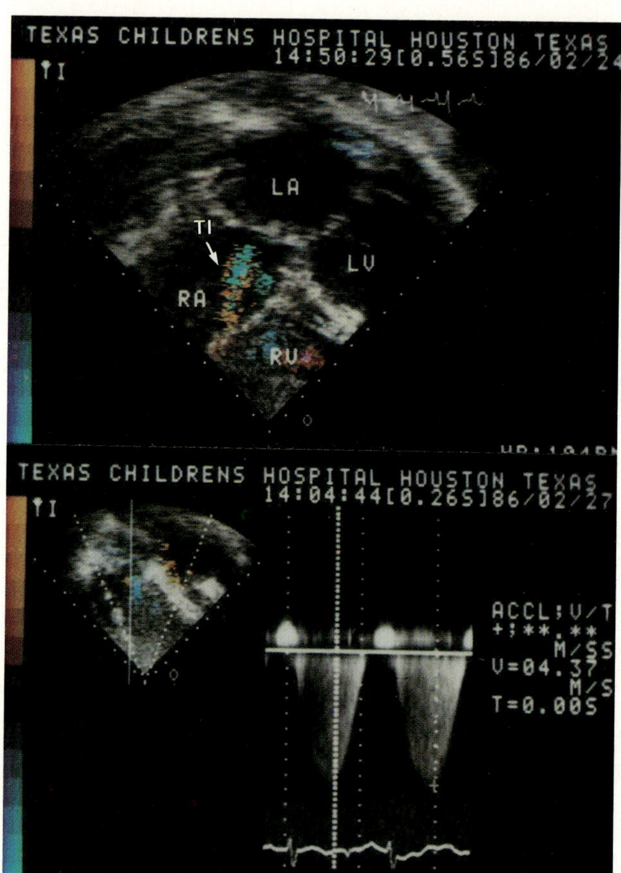

FIGURE 4-16—*Subcostal view demonstrating tricuspid regurgitation oriented toward the atrial septum with variance in the jet. The color display (upper panel) aided the alignment of the continuous-wave Doppler line with the jet (lower panel). The peak velocity of 4.4 meters per second suggested high RV pressure. RV = right ventricle; RA = right atrium; SVC = superior vena cava.*

Superior vena caval flow, inferior vena caval flow, coronary sinus flow, and flow through atrial septal defects occur during systole and could lead to confusion with low-velocity tricuspid regurgitation. These can usually be distinguished with color Doppler by both direction, point of origin, and timing (see Chapter 2).

Tricuspid regurgitation begins with closure of the tricuspid valve. The degree of tricuspid regurgitation is determined by the pressure gradient between the right ventricle and the right atrium, the size of the defect in the closed tricuspid valve, and the compliance of the right atrium and proximal systemic veins. The relationship between pressure drop and peak velocity has been used successfully in adult patients to predict right ventricular pressure in patients with tricuspid regurgitation.[1] However, when the volume of regurgitation is small, it may be difficult to locate the regurgitation jet for quantification of right ventricular pressure. Visualization of the tricuspid regurgitation jet with color Doppler helps in the alignment of the continuous-wave Doppler beam for measurement of peak velocity (Figure 4-16).

Tricuspid regurgitation commonly occurs in patients with congenital heart disease. Tricuspid regurgitation in *Ebstein's anomaly* occurs as a result of gross deformity of the posterior and septal leaflets of the tricuspid valve with adherence to the ventricular wall (see Chapter 6). In addition, pulmonary atresia or stenosis often coexist. Neonates with *pulmonary atresia* and *intact ventricular septum* usually have associated tricuspid regurgitation with right-to-left shunting at the atrial level (see Chapter 6). In addition, transient tricuspid regurgitation occurs in neonates with *persistent pulmonary hypertension*. Visualization of a tricuspid regurgitation jet following repair of *tetralogy of Fallot* with color Doppler flow mapping allows improved estimation of residual right ventricular hypertension by allowing the continuous-wave Doppler beam to be visually aligned with the regurgitation jet (see Chapter 8). Isolated *congenital tricuspid regurgitation* (Figure 4-17) is rare but may occur in the pediatric age range or regurgitation may follow endocarditis.

Conventional Doppler is clearly very sensitive in the *detection* of tricuspid regurgitation.[1,26,27] However, color Doppler appears to be less sensitive to mild degrees of tricuspid regurgitation observed in normal subjects.[10,21] In contrast, Wharton et al.[28] found tricuspid regurgitation more often in normal subjects with color Doppler than with pulsed Doppler, which implies either greater sensitivity and/or less specificity.

The *severity* of tricuspid regurgitation is assessed with conventional Doppler in a manner similar to mitral regurgitation. The regurgitation jet is identified at the tricuspid annulus and traced through the right atrium.[29]

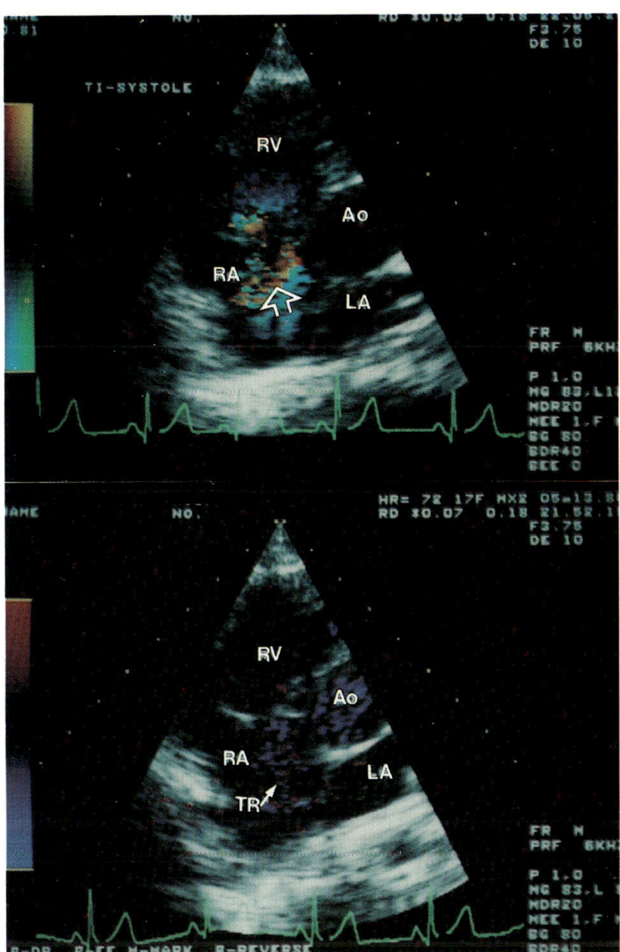

FIGURE 4-17—*Congenital tricuspid valve regurgitation due to dysplasia of the valve in a six-year-old boy. The variance jet (open white arrow) can be seen in short-axis scans (upper panel) and the severity of the regurgitation is confirmed by intensity (power function) mapping (lower panel).*

However, this procedure is complicated by the presence of systolic flow from the superior vena cava, inferior vena cava, and coronary sinus. In addition, the intensity of the jet and the duration during systole have been used as estimates of severity.[1] The measurement of width, length, or area of the color Doppler image of the regurgitation jet promises to be a useful method of assessing regurgitant volume. However, validation is lacking at present. Retrograde systolic flow in the hepatic veins may be seen in normal individuals but is usually transient. With significant tricuspid regurgitation, however, sustained retrograde flow, seen as a red jet in the hepatic veins during systole, may be observed. Intensity color Doppler mapping shows the extent of regurgitation and more closely reflects the volume of regurgitant flow (Figure 4-18).

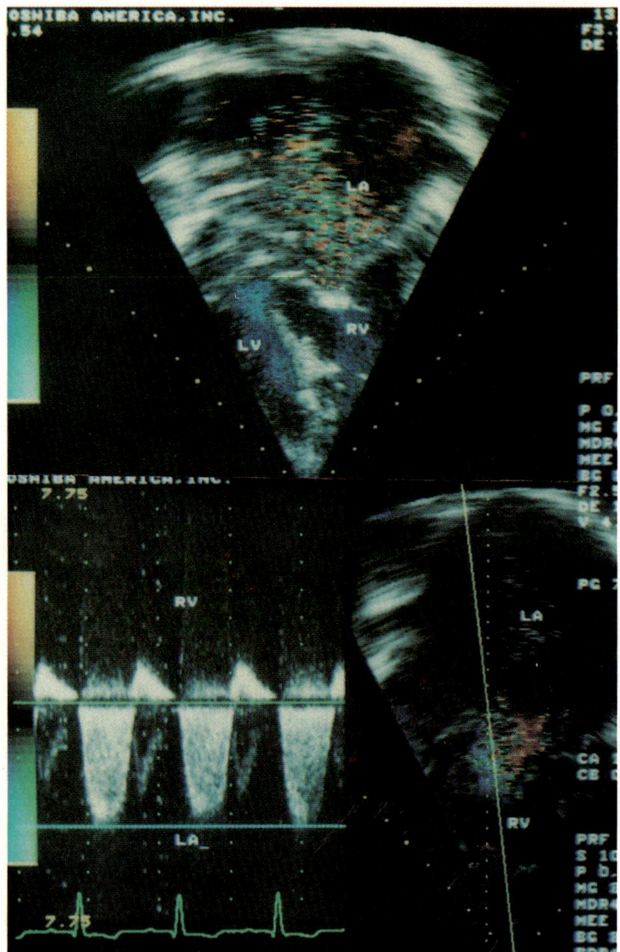

FIGURE 4-18—*Apical four-chamber view in a patient with ventricular inversion (corrected transposition). Left atrioventricular valve regurgitation is visible as a mosaic jet in the massively enlarged left atrium originating from a dysplastic tricuspid (left atrioventricular) valve. RV = right ventricle; LA = left atrium; LV = left ventricle.*

Summary

Color Doppler offers to complement the conventional Doppler examination of both adult and pediatric patients with valvular regurgitation related to congenital heart disease. This method is well suited to the rapid identification of regurgitant jets and may save significant examiner time and improve accuracy when eccentric jets are present. It also appears that color Doppler mapping of regurgitant jets will provide a quantitative estimate of regurgitant volume in mitral and aortic regurgitation. In addition, the direction of the jet of tricuspid regurgitation can be determined which permits better alignment of continuous-wave Doppler cursors for the estimation of right ventricular pressure.

Presently, surgery without catheterization is limited in patients who have congenital defects with valvular regurgitation because it is not possible to grade the severity of the regurgitation. Color Doppler adds confidence to the clinical evaluation of such patients and should allow catheteriaztion to be omitted in many where hemodynamic assessment is the reason for invasive investigation. This method has great potential for the serial evaluation of patients with valvular regurgitation which may improve recognition of deterioration and allow more appropriate timing of medical or surgical intervention.

References

1. Hatle L, Angelsen B: Doppler Ultrasound in Cardiology—Physical Principles and Clinical Applications, 2nd ed. Philadelphia, Lea & Febiger, 1985.
2. Bommer WJ: Basic principles of flow imaging. Echocardiography 2:501-509, 1985.
3. Takenaka K, Dabestani A, Gardin JM, et al: Assessment of the severity of aortic regurgitation by pulsed Doppler abdominal aortic flow pattern. J Am Coll Cardiol 7(2):100A, 1986 (abstr).
4. Ciobanu M, Abbasi AS, Allen M, et al: Pulsed Doppler echocardiography in the diagnosis and estimation of severity of aortic regurgitation. Am J Cardiol 49:339-343, 1982.
5. Chandraratna PAN, Minagoe S, Wade M, et al: Demonstration of regurgitant stream shape and direction in mitral and tricuspid regurgitation by two-dimensional Doppler color flow mapping. J Am Coll Cardiol 5(2):454, 1985.
6. Diebold B, Peronneau P, Blanchard D, et al: Non-invasive quantification of aortic regurgitation by Doppler echocardiography. Br Heart J 49:167-173, 1983.
7. Quinones MA, Young JB, Waggoner AD, et al: Assessment of pulsed Doppler echocardiography in detection and quantification of aortic and mitral regurgitation. Br Heart J 44:612-620, 1980.
8. Sequiera RF, Watt I: Assessment of aortic regurgitation by transcutaneous aortovelography. Br Heart J 39:929-930, 1977.
9. Rokey R, Sterling LL, Zoghibi WA, et al: Determination of regurgitant fraction in isolated mitral or aortic regurgitation by pulsed Doppler two-dimensional echocardiography. J Am Coll Cardiol 7(6):1263-1271, 1986.
10. Yock PG, Segal J, Teirstein PS, et al: Doppler color flow mapping: Utility in valvular regurgitation. Circulation 70(Suppl II):II-38, 1984 (abstr).
11. Asaka T, Yoshikawa J, Yoshida K, et al: Sensitivity and specificity of real-time two-dimensional Doppler flow imaging system in the detection of valvular regurgitation. Circulation 70(Suppl II):II-38, 1984 (abstr).
12. Byard CE, Perry GJ, Roitman DI, et al: Quantitative assessment of aortic regurgitation by color Doppler. Circulation 72(4):III-146, 1985 (abstr).
13. Omoto R, Yokote Y, Takamoto S, et al: The development of real-time two-dimensional Doppler echocardiography and its clinical significance in acquired valvular diseases. Jpn Heart J, 25:325-340, 1984.
14. Switzer DF, Nanda NC: Color Doppler evaluation of valvular regurgitation. Echocardiography 2,533-543, 1985.

15. Perry GJ, Helmcke F, Nanda NC: Color Doppler assessment of aortic regurgitation in two orthogonal planes. J Am Coll Cardiol 7:101A, 1986 (abstr).
16. Pearlman AS, Otto CM, Janko CL, Reamer RP: Direction and width of aortic regurgitant jets: Assessment by Doppler color flow mapping. J Am Coll Cardiol 7:100A, 1986 (abstr).
17. Brouchard A, Yock PG, Schiller NB, et al: Quantitation of chronic aortic regurgitation using color Doppler flow mapping. Circulation 72(Suppl III):III-100, 1985 (abstr).
18. Takao S, Miyatake K, Isumi S, et al: Physiological pulmonary regurgitation detected by the Doppler technique and its differential diagnosis. J Am Coll Cardiol 5:499, 1985.
19. Yock PG, Naasz C, Schnittger I, Popp RL: Doppler tricuspid and pulmonic regurgitation in normals: Is it real? Circulation 70(Suppl II):II-40, 1984 (abstr).
20. Recusani F, Valdes-Cruz L, Dalton N, et al: Tricuspid and pulmonary regurgitation and right heart flow patterns in normals: Studies using color coded flow mapping and pulsed Doppler. Circulation 72(Suppl III):III-307, 1985 (abstr).
21. Braunwald E: Heart Disease: A Textbook of Cardiovascular Medicine, 2nd ed. Philadelphia, WB Saunders Co, 1984, p 1078.
22. Abbasi AS, Allen MW, Decristofaro D, Ungar I: Detection and estimation of the degree of mitral regurgitation by range gated pulsed Doppler echocardiography. Circulation 61:143-147, 1980.
23. Bommer WJ, Rebeck KF, Laviola S, et al: Real-time two dimensional flow imaging: Detection and semiquantification of valvular and congenital heart disease. Circulation 70(Suppl II):II-38, 1984 (abstr).
24. Saenz CB, Deumite J, Roitman DI, et al: Limitations of color Doppler in quantitative assessment of mitral regurgitation. Circulation 72(Suppl III):III-99, 1985 (abstr).
25. Yock PG, Popp RL: Noninvasive estimation of right ventricular systolic pressure by Doppler ultrasound in patients with tricuspid regurgitation. Circulation 70:657-662, 1984.
26. Stevenson JG, Kawabori I, Guntheroth W: Validation of Doppler diagnosis of tricuspid regurgitation. Circulation 64(Suppl IV):IV-255, 1981 (abstr).
27. Wharton JM, NeSmith JW, Shaw MC: Comparison of conventional Doppler and Doppler color flow mapping of the right atrium in normal volunteers. Circulation 72 (Suppl III):III-98, 1985 (abstr).
28. Miyatake K, Okamoto M, Kinoshita N, et al: Evaluation of tricuspid regurgitation by pulsed Doppler and two-dimensional echocardiography. Circulation 66:777-784, 1982.

Chapter 5

Left-to-Right Shunts

Achi Ludomirsky, M.D., and James C. Huhta, M.D.

Left-to-right shunts are the most frequently encountered hemodynamic abnormality due to a congenital cardiac defect. They may cause serious symptoms during the first months of life as the result of the drop in right ventricular pressure below the level of the left ventricle after birth. Left-to-right shunting causes volume overload of the pulmonary system and the left heart. Two-dimensional echocardiography has been shown to be of great use in the detection of various shunt lesions. It is now widely accepted that imaging of the ventricular septum, atrial septum, aorta, and the pulmonary artery in multiple views can detect abnormal congenital communications.[1] Using the pulsed and continuous-wave Doppler technique, intracardiac shunt flow and pressure gradient can also be analyzed by these methods.[2] Direct detection of shunt flows using pulsed and continuous-wave Doppler combined with imaging by two-dimensional echocardiography is available but requires a significant amount of time in the mapping of normal signals at various sites in the cardiac chambers.[3] Contrast echocardiography with peripheral injection of contrast medium was the only noninvasive method for direct visualization of intracardiac shunts. Color Doppler is useful in the detection of shunt flow velocity and may provide semiquantitive measurements of flow across a shunt and can be used for detection of residual shunts after surgical intervention.[4]

Atrial Septal Defects

Atrial septal defects are best visualized in subcostal scans supplemented by apical four-chamber and parasternal views and, because a defect rather than a structure is being scanned, these same views optimize the blood flow velocity in the defect. Doppler in the diagnosis of atrial septal defects is added to imaging to determine whether or not there is flow across the atrial septum.[2] In the case of dropout in the two-dimensional echocardiography imaging, sampling with pulsed Doppler in the dropout area should solve this problem. However, the presence of left-to-right shunt through a "patent foramen ovale" in neonates is common when left atrial pressure is elevated, such as with a ventricular septal defect, and does not necessarily mean that an atrial septal defect will be present at an older age.

Pulsed Doppler has been shown to have an excellent sensitivity and specificity for the diagnosis of atrial septal defect.[5] Doppler evaluation is useful for detection of other flow disturbances occurring in the right atrium such as might be seen with partial anomalous venous return or tricuspid regurgitation. Doppler can also be used in the determination of flow direction and the magnitude of atrial septal defect shunts.

Color Doppler is useful in evaluating atrial septal defects. Suzuki et al. evaluated the noninvasive detection of shunt flow across an atrial septum using color Doppler and contrast echocardiography.[6] They found that color Doppler increased the sensitivity over contrast echocardiography for detecting left-to-right shunts at the atrial level in adults from 50 percent to 70 percent; however, the specificity was slightly less in color Doppler (90 percent) than in contrast echocardiography (100 percent). Color Doppler will easily differentiate between the three types of atrial septal defects by detecting the origin of the jet from the left atrium into the right atrium or into the superior caval-right atrial junction with sinus venosus atrial septal defects. The interatrial shunt occurs in late systole and early diastole with secundum ASD. Because of the low velocity across the lesion, the jet is depicted as a homogeneous red pattern starting at the left atrial side of the defect and passing through the lesion into the right atrium (Figure 5-1). The parasternal short axis is also useful to detect the presence of an interatrial communication by color Doppler (Figure 5-2). Pulsed Doppler confirms that the left-to-right shunt is occurring in late systole and early diastole (Figure 5-3). In cases of a high-pressure gradient between the left and the right atrium, the flow velocity can alias (Figure 5-4). When there is a restrictive interatrial communication and not

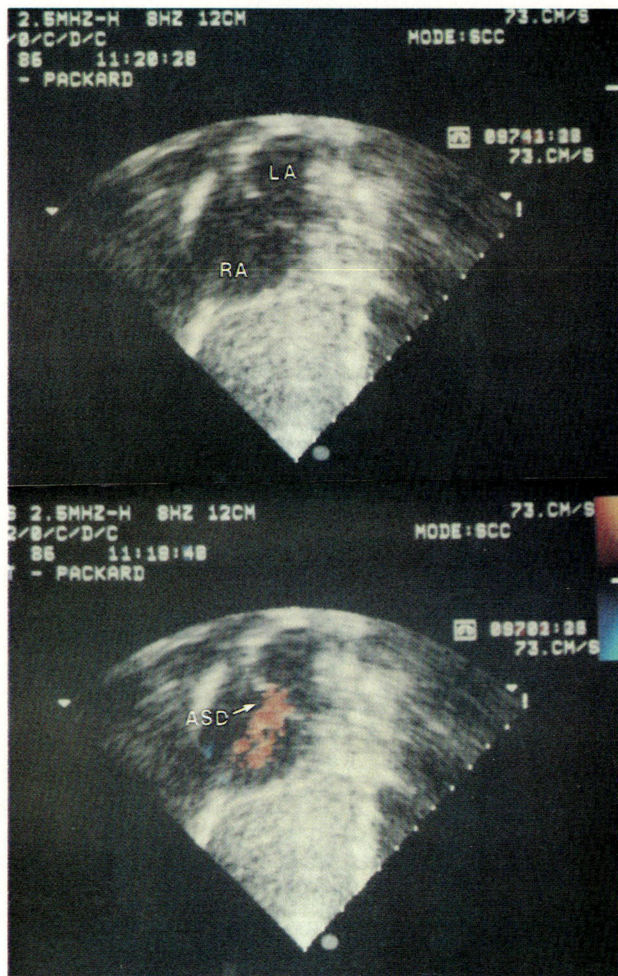

FIGURE 5-1—*Color Doppler in a two-year-old boy with a secundum ASD. A subcostal four-chamber view shows the left atrium (LA) and the right atrium (RA) in cross-section. Two-dimensional imaging (upper panel) shows a large secundum ASD. The jet is depicted in red (lower panel) shunting from the left atrium into the right atrium during late systole and early diastole. ASD = atrial septal defect.*

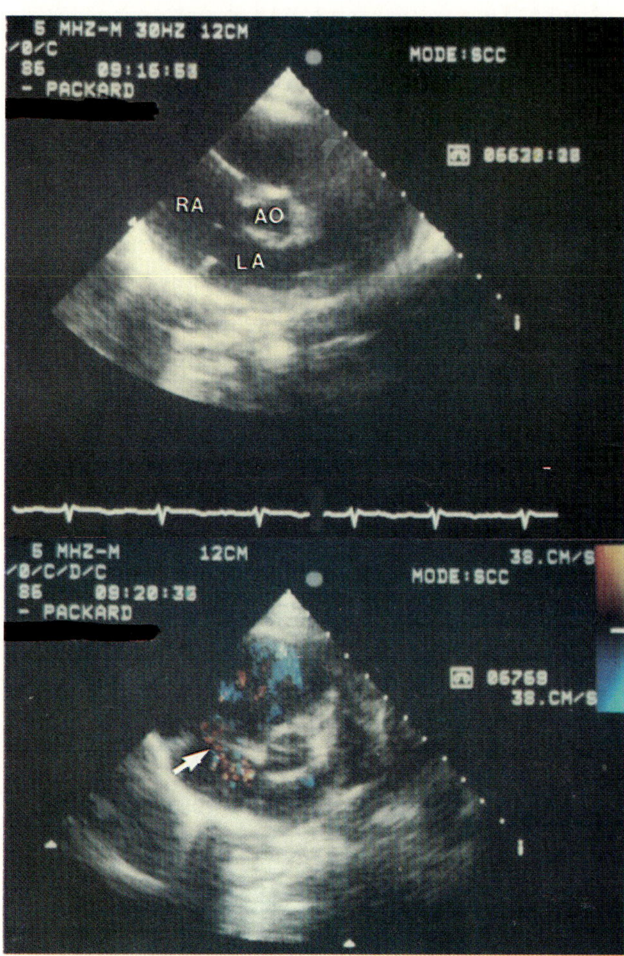

FIGURE 5-2—*Parasternal short-axis of a three-year-old child with secundum ASD (upper panel). Color Doppler (lower panel) indicates turbulence across the interatrial septum as seen by a mosaic pattern in the right atrium proximal to the tricuspid valve (arrow). AO = aorta; LA = left atrium; RA = right atrium.*

necessarily a congenital defect, the peak velocity on Doppler occurs in mid-systole and flow does not continue into diastole (compare Figures 5-4 and 5-3). High-velocity aliasing occurs with significant obstruction at the fossa ovalis, as in mitral atresia (Figure 5-5, upper panel).

In the diagnosis of atrial septal defect, color Doppler is important for differentiating between normal right superior vena cava flow into the right atrium and abnormal left-to-right shunting across the atrial septum (Figure 5-4). The normal right SVC shunt is directed parallel and close to the lateral wall, while the ASD jet is directed toward the tricuspid valve.

The efficacy of balloon atrial septostomy in a transposition of the great arteries, anomalous venous return, and mitral atresia is well known. Color Doppler provides a tool for noninvasive evaluation of this procedure. In conclusion, color Doppler is useful in the detection of atrial septal defects, characterization of the flow, and rough estimates of the magnitude of left-to-right shunt in this level. Mapping of the jet in the right atrium may help detection of the flow jet for quantitation of interatrial pressure gradient with pulsed and continuous-wave Doppler when there is obstruction (Figure 5-5).

Ventricular Septal Defects

The principal factors in detection of ventricular septal defects appear to be the location, size, and relative

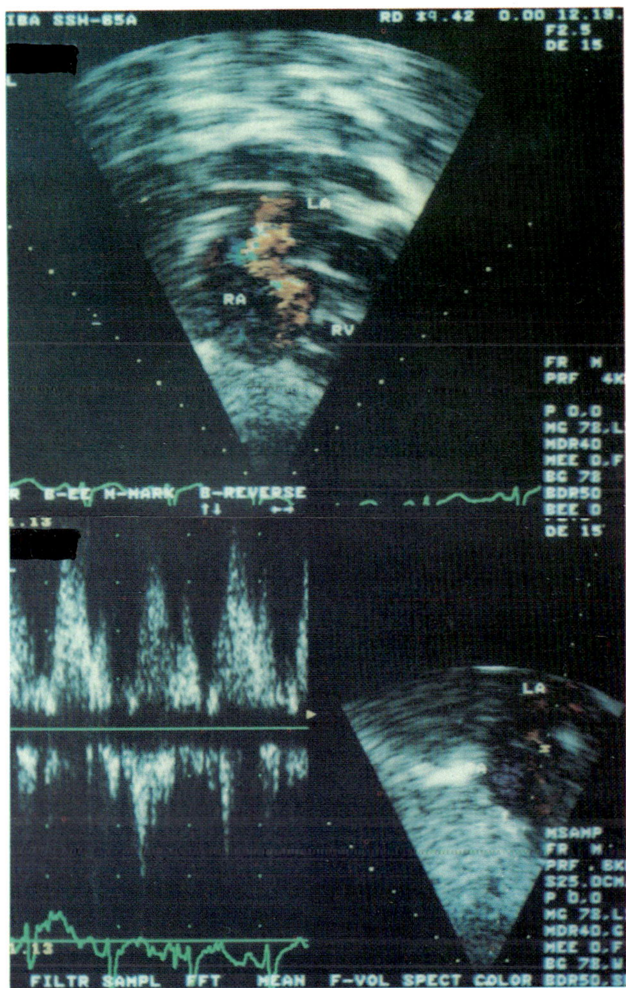

FIGURE 5-3—*A modified subcostal four-chamber view of a baby with a large left-to-right shunt across a secundum atrial defect (ASD). The flow can be seen in the right atrium filling a significant portion of this chamber during diastole. Confirmation of the diagnosis of the left-to-right shunt using pulsed Doppler with the beam aligned parallel to the ASD jet is shown in the lower panel. LA = left atrium; RA = right atrium; RV = right ventricle.*

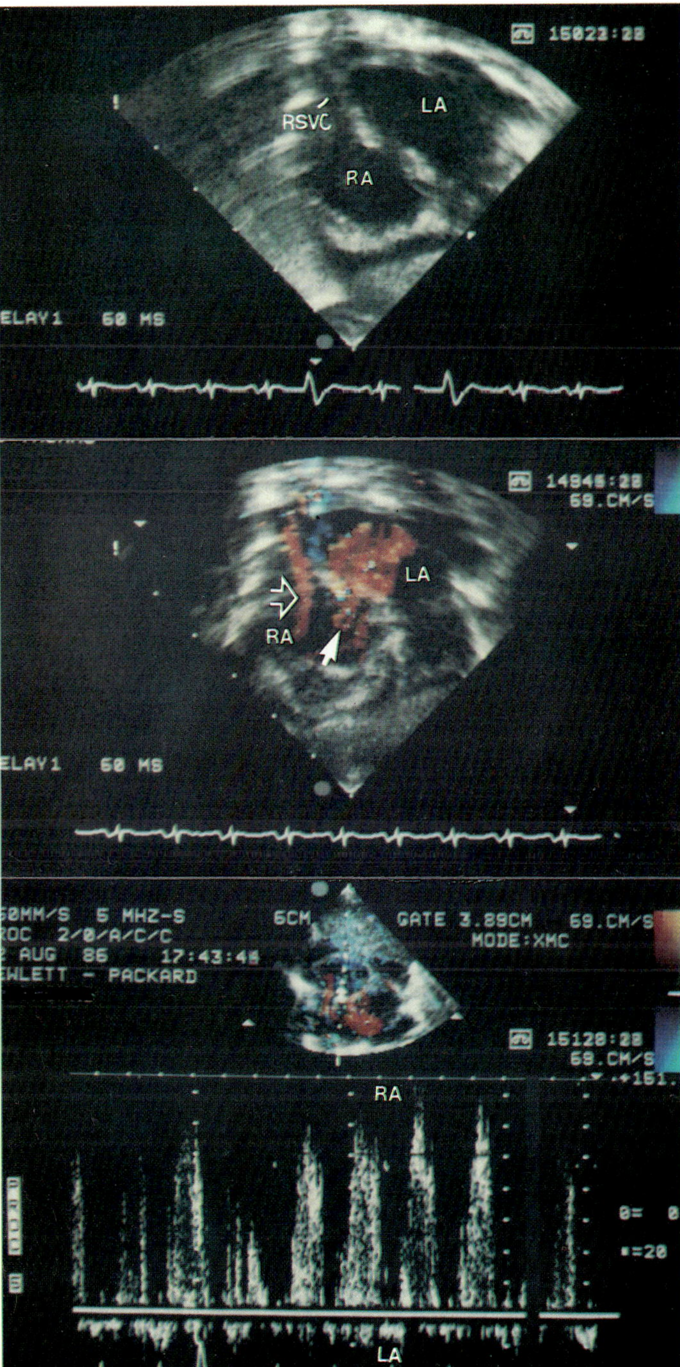

FIGURE 5-4—*Subcostal view of a one-month-old baby with a stretched patent foramen ovale and left atrial hypertension due to a ventricular septal defect. Different flows in the right atrium could cause difficulty in the detection of the left-to-right atrial shunt jet. Color Doppler easily differentiates between the normal superior caval flow intensity jet into the right atrium (open arrow) and shunt jet from left atrium to right atrium (closed arrow) (middle panel). Sampling with pulsed Doppler in the jet confirms the diagnosis and the presence of interatrial pressure gradient (lower panel). LA = left atrium; RA = right atrium; RSVC =* right superior vena cava.

ventricular pressures as well as the directions of blood flow. The ventricular septal defects are usually classified as perimembraneous, muscular, or outlet, and the relationships to other intracardiac structures are then described. Detection of early aneurysm formation and involvement of the tricuspid valve tissue in diminishing the size of the VSD is important in the evaluation of the natural history of this defect. A jet directed superiorly toward the aortic valve may predispose to aortic insufficiency. In the two-dimensional echocardiographic image, the VSD appears as a distinct interruption of the normal continuity of the intraventricular septum. The

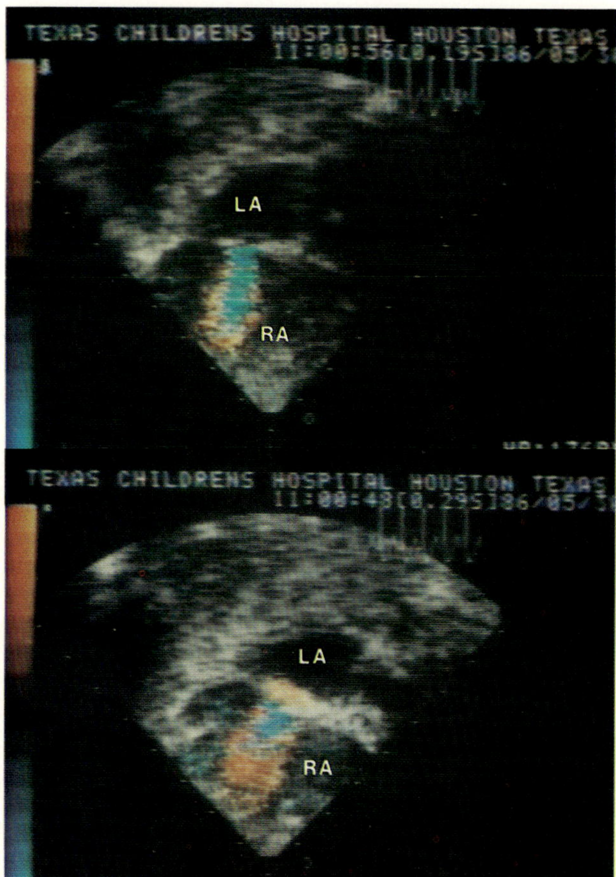

FIGURE 5-5—*Color Doppler of the atrial septum before and after balloon atrial septostomy. This two-month-old baby with mitral atresia had a restrictive defect before septostomy (upper panel). The high flow velocities across the atrial septum caused complete color reversal of the jet toward the transducer. The jet is depicted in blue with a red-orange vortex indicating turbulence in this area. Immediately after the procedure (lower panel), the area occupied by this jet was enlarged and the aliasing reached only the upper third of the right atrium, indicating a decrease of flow velocity. LA = left atrium; RA = right atrium.*

usual short- and long-axis views from the parasternal position are best for Doppler. The apical four-chamber and subcostal four-chamber views successfully characterize the different types of ventricular septal defect.[1]

Pulsed Doppler echocardiography has been used to detect the presence of flow disturbances within the heart caused by a ventricular septal defect. Stevenson et al. used pulsed Doppler to evaluate residual ventricular septal defect patches in a postoperative study.[3] This work confirmed the presence of left-to-right shunting that occurred in the early postoperative period following patch repair of ventricular septal defect. The feasibility of noninvasive ventricular septal defect pressure gradient measurement by continuous-wave Doppler[7] has been demonstrated recently. Peak right ventricular systolic pressure can be estimated and measurement of the pulmonary-to-systemic flow ratio as an indicator of shunt magnitude is possible using Doppler.[8,9] Shunt size estimates are useful for assessing pulmonary resistance. Ortiz et al. has underlined one of the most useful applications of color Doppler in the identification and localization of ventricular septal defects.[10]

We studied the sensitivity and specificity for detection of isolated and multiple ventricular septal defect using two-dimensional color Doppler and regular two-dimensional echocardiography. In the detection of multiple ventricular septal defect, the sensitivity of color Doppler was 72 percent and that of two-dimensional and Doppler was only 38 percent (100 percent specificity in both). It was concluded that color Doppler is useful for the detection of ventricular septal defects and has higher sensitivity than two-dimensional and Doppler for multiple ventricular septal defects.[11]

Color Doppler may be used in the localization of small defects and to assess the direction of the shunt flow. As in stenotic lesions, color Doppler serves as a guideline for alignment of the continuous-wave Doppler beam for desirable spectral displays. Using the electrocardiographic gating mode provides the detection of different jet directions during systole and diastole, especially in patients with elevated right ventricular pressure and right-to-left shunting. Figure 5-6 shows a typical appearance of VSD by color Doppler in the long and short parasternal views of a patient with a restrictive defect. During systole, a jet directed from the left ventricle to the right ventricle across the interventricular septum is identified by the turbulence in this area in a jet that has a mosaic pattern. Pulsed and continuous-wave Doppler enhance the diagnosis of ventricular septal defect. Figure 5-7 shows the usefulness of color flow mapping in the alignment of the continuous-wave Doppler beam with the flow velocity jet. From the parasternal long axis with the jet directed from the left ventricle in the right ventricle toward the transducer, the spectral display of the continuous-wave Doppler has a positive deflection toward the transducer. Figure 5-8 shows the short-axis view of the same patient using directed continuous-wave for display.

M-mode echocardiography is useful for accurate measurement of the ventricular dimension in VSD. When color Doppler is used in conjunction with M-mode, precise timing of the shunt is possible (Figure 5-9).

Apical and subcostal four-chamber views are of help in the detection of *perimembranous ventricular septal defect* (Figure 5-10). A mosaic pattern in the area of ventricular septal defect occurs because of turbulence in this region. The perimembranous jets shown in the apical

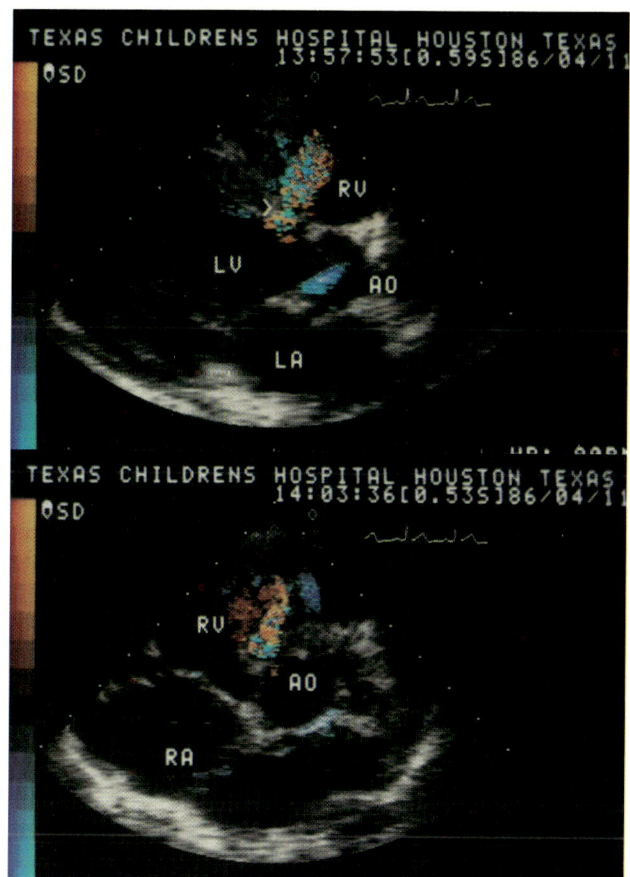

FIGURE 5-6—*Parasternal long- and short-axis views of a five-year-old with perimembranous VSD (upper panel). In the long-axis display , the color jet with mosaic pattern is seen in the right ventricle. The same turbulent jet across the perimembranous area is seen in the lower panel in the short-axis view. Both still frames were taken in systole (electrocardiographic gating). Ao = aorta; LA = left atrium; LV = left ventricle; RV = right ventricle; VSD = ventricular septal defect.*

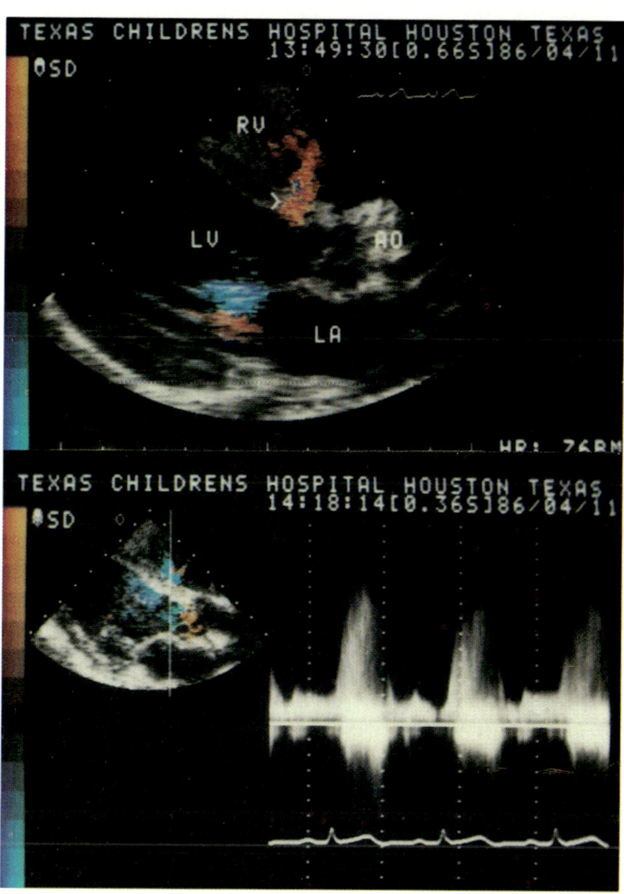

FIGURE 5-7—*The parasternal long-axis of a two-year-old patient with perimembranous VSD. The diagnosis was confirmed with color Doppler (upper panel) and by continuous-wave Doppler (lower panel). Accurate parallel alignment of the continuous-wave beam and the VSD jet achieved the desirable spectral display. Ao = aorta; LA = left atrium; LV = left ventricle; RV = right ventricle.*

and subcostal four-chamber view are aimed toward the transducer and depicted as red jets in the right ventricle (Figure 5-11).

Careful scanning of the ventricular septum in the parasternal short-axis and in the apical four-chamber view is necessary for the detection of *muscular defects*. Figure 5-12 shows the color flow display of a patient with a large muscular ventricular septal defect. The perimembranous region appears to be intact but color Doppler turbulence may radiate to the outflow region of the right ventricle and make the diagnosis of two defects difficult from the parasternal approach.

The red blood cell velocity crossing the ventricular septal defect is proportional to the pressure gradient between the two ventricles. In most cases high-velocity aliasing occurs and aids the detection of small muscular defects (Figure 5-13). In cases of equal-pressure ventricles, either blue jets or a mosaic pattern can be seen in systole as a reflection of lower velocity in the muscular defect (compare Figures 5-14 and 5-15).

Careful scanning of the ventricular septum in the apical four-chamber view is necessary for the detection of small and/or additional ventricular septal defects in the muscular septum. In such defects the transeptal flow jet is predominately away from the transducer and coded blue, and can be separated from the diastolic inflow in the opposite direction which appears as a red color coded flow within the right ventricle. In a case of multiple ventricular septal defect, two or more jets coded blue will be seen arising from the inferior (apical) septum of the right ventricle (Figure 5-16).

Large shunts across the ventricular septal defect increase the pulmonary blood flow. As shown in Figure

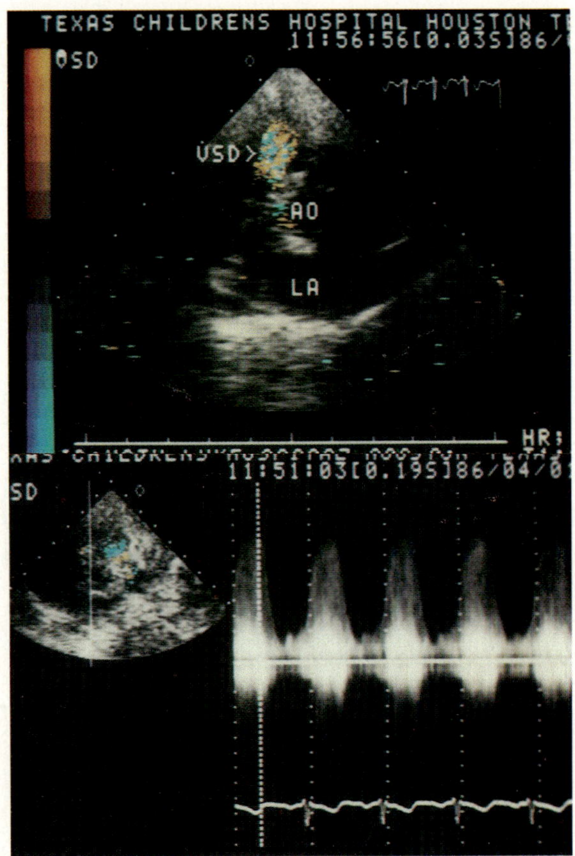

FIGURE 5-8—*Parasternal short-axis of a three-year-old boy with a small perimembranous ventricular septal defect (VSD). The color Doppler display showed a variance jet from the perimembranous area into the right ventricle (upper panel). The continuous-wave Dopler evaluation for hemodynamic prediction of pressure gradient across the defect showed a velocity of 3.5 meters per second or an instantaneous gradient of 50 mm-Hg. Ao = aorta; LA = left atrium.*

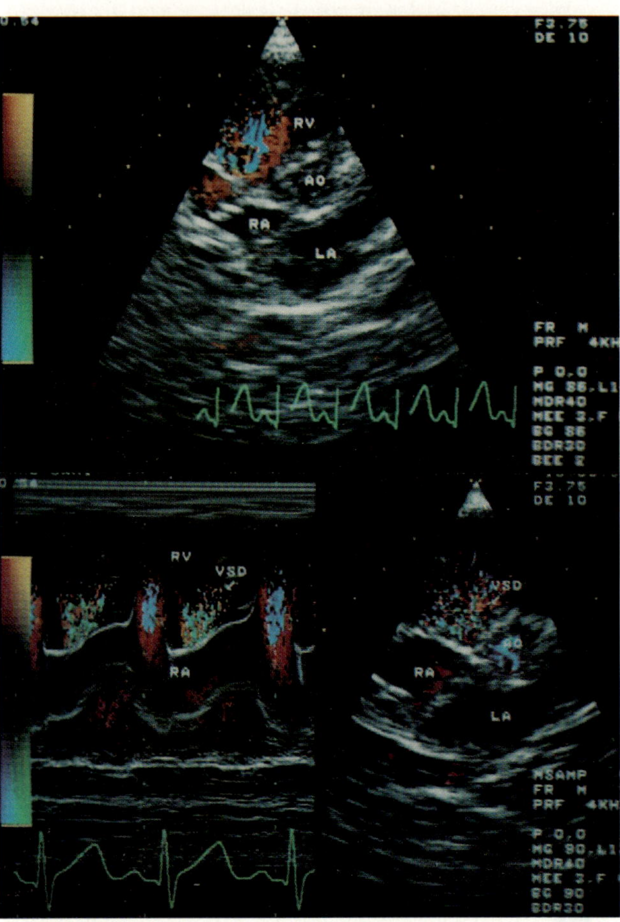

FIGURE 5-9—*Parasternal short-axis in a five-year-old boy with a small perimembranous ventricular septal defect (VSD). A frame gated in systole shows a variance jet in the right ventricle (upper panel) on color display. The M-mode color display (lower panel) shows the VSD jet confined to systole. AO = aorta; LA = left atrium; LV = left ventricle; RA = right atrium; RV = right ventricle.*

5-17 (upper panel), the color flow area across the pulmonary valve is widened compared to the normal flow with aliasing. If the shunt is not large because of severe pulmonary hypertension (Eisenmenger's syndrome), then bidirectional shunt will be present on color Doppler (Figure 5-17, lower panel). Studies of the timing of VSD shunting are best performed using M-mode color Doppler echocardiography (Figure 5-18).

In conclusion, color Doppler is useful for the detection of ventricular septal defects and has greater sensitivity than two-dimensional and Doppler echocardiography for multiple ventricular septal defects. The contribution of color Doppler appears to be its ability to detect additional small and multiple septal defects as well as aiding in the determination of the direction of the jet.

Atrioventricular Canal Defects

Two-dimensional echocardiography is the best noninvasive imaging tool for visualization of the atrial and ventricular septae. The anatomy of atrioventricular canal defects is best imaged from the apical or subcostal four-chamber views. The essential features of AV canal defect are absence of the atrioventricular septum and abnormal development of the atrioventricular valves. Two-dimensional echocardiography accurately visualizes the AV valve tissue and the support appartus. Studies have shown that this noninvasive modality is superior to angiography in characterization of AV valve leaflet abnormalities.[12] Partial, intermediate, and complete forms of AV canal defect differ principally in the attachments of the valves to the septum and the size of the interventricu-

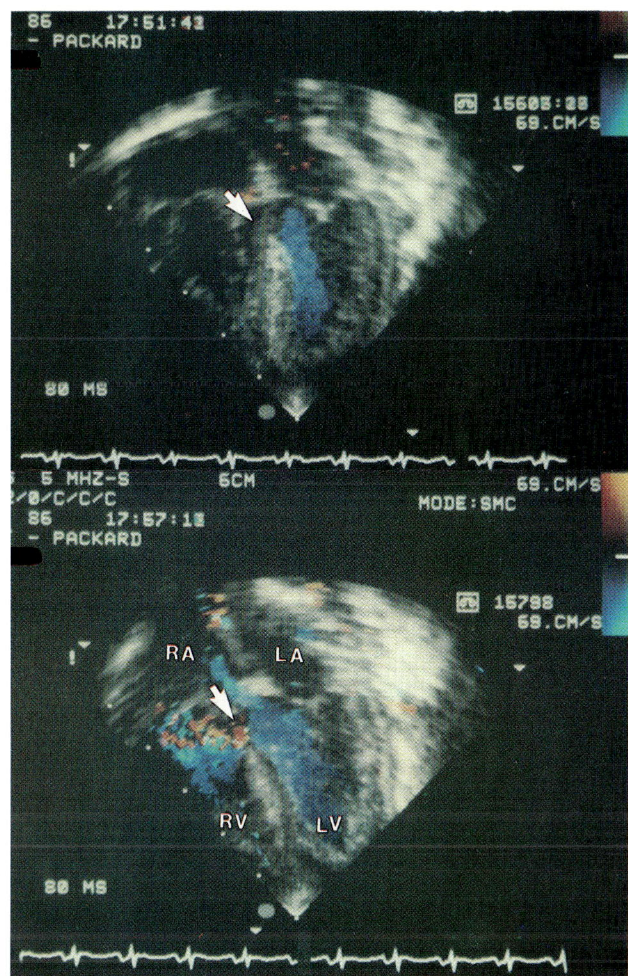

FIGURE 5-10—*Apical four-chamber view of a six-year-old girl with perimembranous ventricular septal defect (arrow in both panels). Angulation of the transducer from a straight four-chamber view (upper panel) to a more subcostal projection shows the improvement in velocity detection in the VSD and variance in the jet. LA = left atrium; LV = left ventricle; RA = right atrium; RV = right ventricle.*

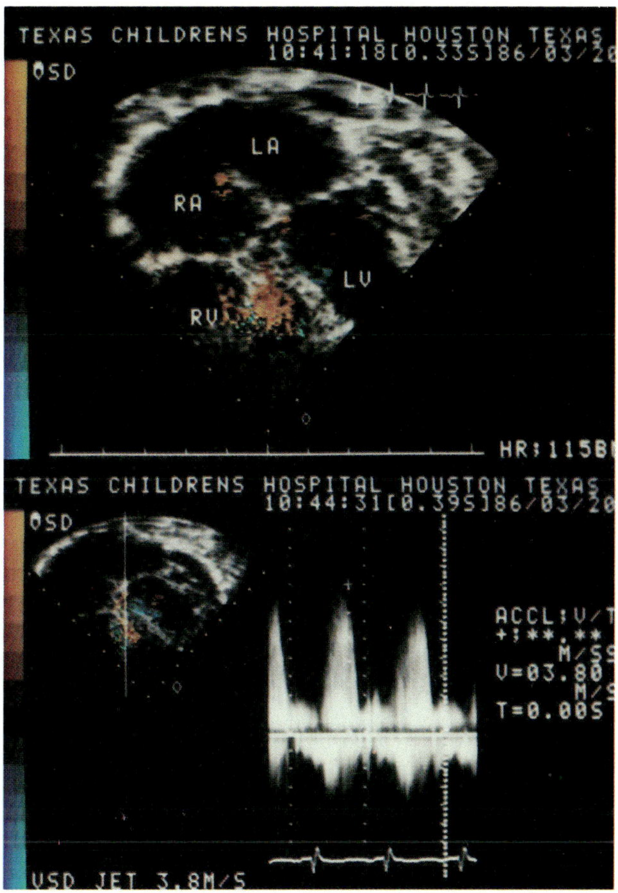

FIGURE 5-11—*Apical four-chamber view of a three-year-old girl with restrictive interventricular septal defect. The jet from a perimembranous defect is streaming toward the right ventricular (RV) apex and the transducer, and has a red-orange appearance (upper panel). Continuous-wave Doppler aligned with the jet confirms the diagnosis of restrictive VSD with a pressure gradient between the two ventricles of 57 mmHg. LA = left atrium; LV = left ventricle; RA = right atrium.*

lar communication. Several important anatomical details should be defined: (1) the amount of the common AV valve tissue that is present, (2) the function of the AV valves, (3) left ventricular or right ventricular outflow obstruction, (4) attachment of the valve chordae to the ventricular septum, and (5) additional systemic venous or pulmonary venous anomalies.

In the typical partial AVC defect there are separate atrioventricular orifices so that the tricuspid and mitral valves are attached at the same level. In the region normally occupied by the AV septum there is an atrial septal defect without an intraventricular communication. Attachment of the tricuspid and mitral valves to the crest of the septum is displaced inferiorly and is at the same level without any ventricular component of the defect. Another feature of primum ASD is the associated cleft mitral valve which is well visualized in the apical four-chamber and parasternal short-axis views.

Complete AV canal defects are characterized by the presence of a common atrioventricular orifice usually consisting of four or five leaflets and a large interventricular communication. The atrial septal defect component is usually very large.[13]

Doppler echocardiography has complemented two-dimensional echocardiographic imaging for hemodynamic evaluation of these patients. Pulsed and continuous-wave Doppler is used for semiquantitation of the AV valve regurgitation. Left-to-right or right-to-left shunts can be detected; however, there are frequently multiple

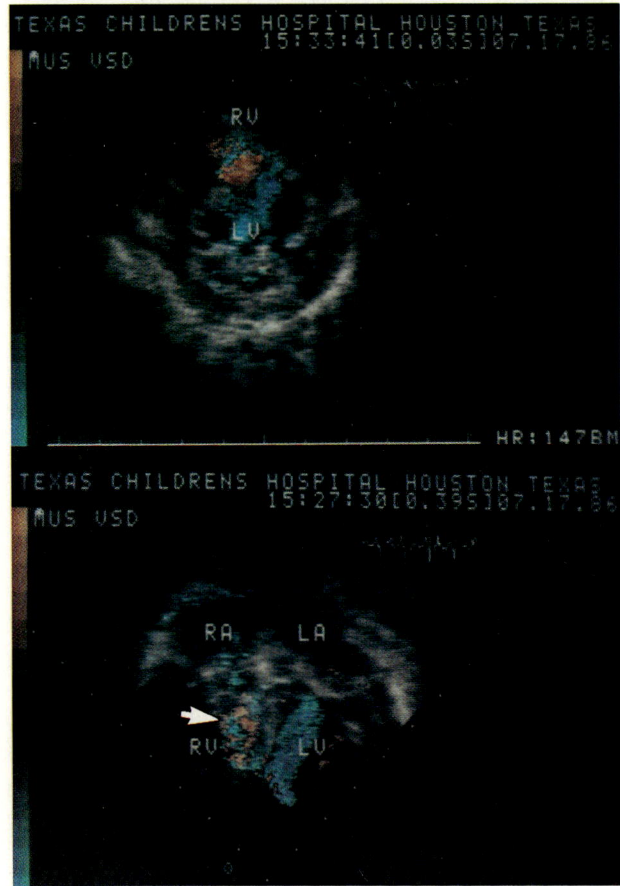

FIGURE 5-12—*Parasternal short-axis (upper panel) and apical four-chamber view (lower panel) of a patient with a large muscular ventricular septal defect. A large red jet with variance arising from the left ventricle across the defect in the mid-trabecular septum marks the site of shunting. The same patient scanned from the apical four-chamber view showed a large jet arising from the muscular septum of the left ventricle (LV) toward the right ventricle (RV) depicted as a mosaic pattern (arrow). LA = left atrium; RA = right atrium.*

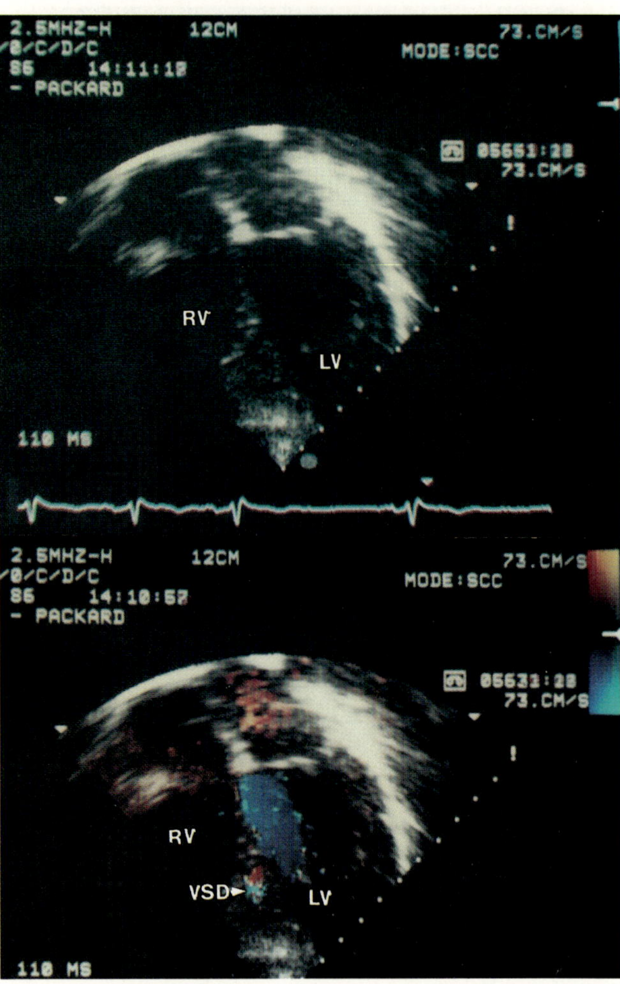

FIGURE 5-13—*Apical four-chamber view of a three-year-old with a restrictive muscular ventricular septal defect (VSD). The jet is aliasing and is depicted as red with a mosaic pattern near the apex. LV = left ventricle; RV = right ventricle.*

jets of flow velocity in the heart, which can make the pulsed Doppler examination difficult.[2]

Color flow mapping in AV canal defects provides superior information about jet direction and valvular regurgitation.[14] Both partial and complete forms have a color Doppler appearance of bilateral ventricular filling in diastole (Figure 5-19). The very high velocity jet of left ventricle to right atrium shunt through the cleft valve is another feature of both lesions (Figure 5-20). The most prominent feature of partial AV canal defect is the interatrial shunting which starts in late systole and continues into late diastole (Figure 5-21). Separation of tricuspid valve (right-sided portion of the AV valve) regurgitation can be accomplished using continuous-wave Doppler directed by color Doppler and confirms that the right ventricular pressure is low (Figure 5-22). Further work is necessary to define the ability of color Doppler to quantitate the degree of valvular regurgitation in this complex congenital cardiac lesion.

Patent Ductus Arteriosus

A patent ductus arteriosus (PDA) is a persistent communication by a muscular tube between the aorta and the pulmonary artery. This communication normally closes within days after birth and persistence leads to left-to-right shunt. Such a defect may present in an infant with congestive heart failure or in an asymptomatic adult. Color Doppler makes the recognition of a patent/persistent ductus arteriosus relatively straightforward if an adequate parasternal or suprasternal window can be obtained which aligns the ductal jet with the ultasound beam. When the shunt through the PDA is large, one

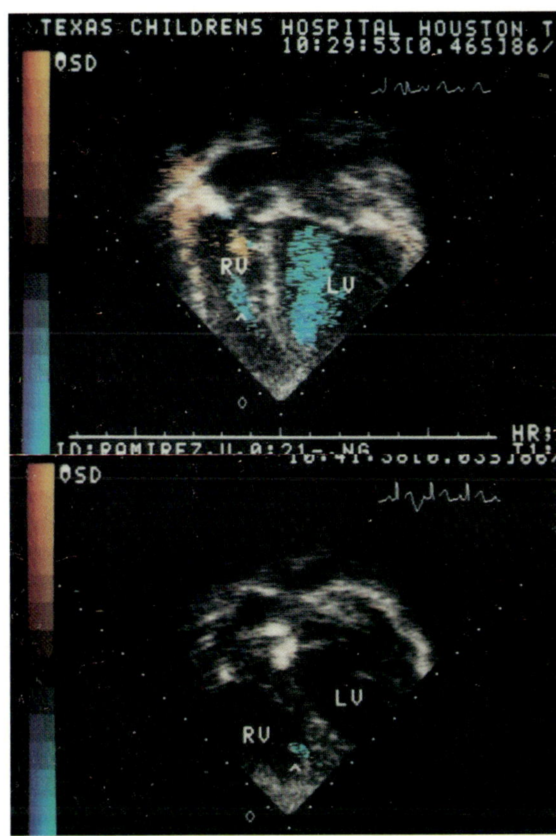

FIGURE 5-14—*Apical four-chamber view of a patient with a low-velocity jet across the muscular ventricular septum (arrows): early systole (upper panel) and later in systole (lower panel). There is a homogeneous blue jet away from the transducer indicative of a defect in the ventricular septum. LV = left ventricle; RV = right ventricle.*

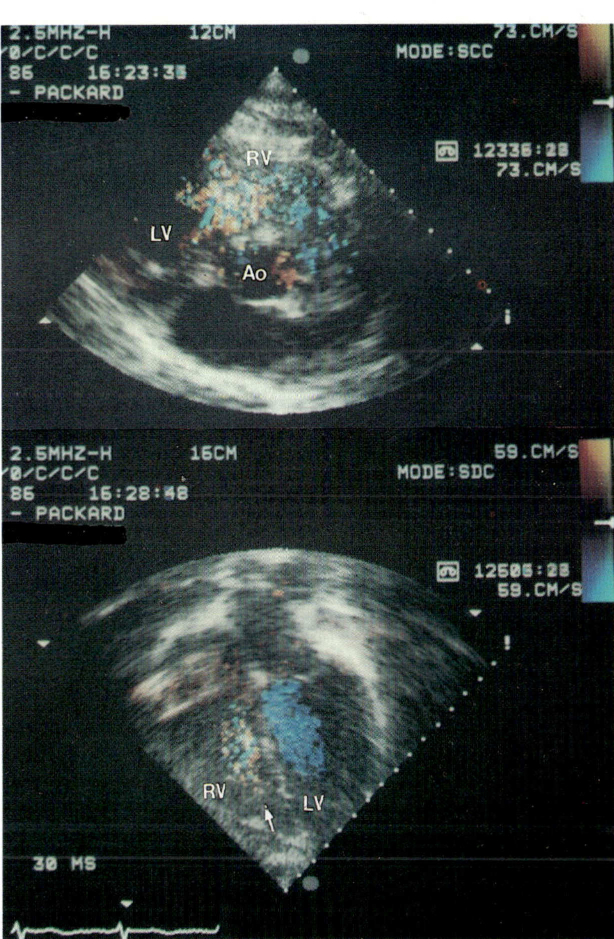

FIGURE 5-15—*Parasternal short-axis and apical four-chamber views of a patient with a large apical ventricular septal defect and pulmonary hypertension. In the upper panel, the jet is depicted in a mosaic pattern reflective of the turbulence in this area. The apical four-chamber view helps identify the origin of this jet near the apex of the heart (arrow). Ao = aorta; LV = left ventricle; RV = right ventricle.*

finds diastolic reversal of descending aortic flow, diastolic runoff in the left pulmonary artery, and frequently pulmonary insufficiency. Continuous-wave Doppler can be used for detection of patent ductus arteriosus and has the added benefit of being able to quantify the ductal gradient using the Bernoulli equation (Figure 5-23). By converting each velocity point (V) to a pressure gradient ($4\ V^2$), the peak and mean gradients can be determined quantitatively.

The angle of left-to-right shunt from a PDA depends on many factors, the most important of which is how much constriction is present. A constricted PDA tends to be directed more inferiorly than one that is wide open. The continuous-wave Doppler line can then be aligned with the jet (Figure 5-24). A velocity of nearly 4 meters per second (Figures 5-24 and 5-25) virtually excludes severe pulmonary hypertension.

In *pulmonary atresia*, the ductus may be the sole supply of pulmonary blood flow. The location of a patent ductus in pulmonary atresia is typically under the arch (Figure 5-26). The location and patency of a ductus have importance in the preoperative evaluation of infants with reduced pulmonary blood flow since many will undergo surgery without catheterization.

Patent ductus arteriosus in a *premature* infant can be a serious problem and excluding PDA in such babies has great clinical importance (Figure 5-27). A patent ductus of only 1 or 2 millimeters in diameter can be significant in a very premature neonate. The projection for imaging with Doppler is a high parasternal or suprasternal view with imaging of the left pulmonary artery and the descending aorta (Figure 5-28). Because of limited imaging capability in the neonate who weighs under 1,000 grams, Doppler is necessary for the diagnosis and may give some clues about the amount of flow through the ductus arteriosus.[15]

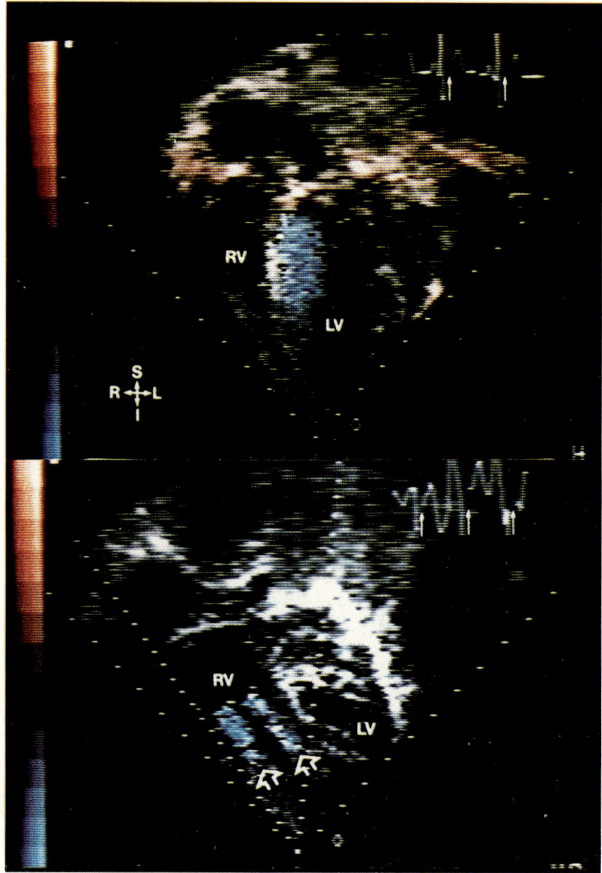

FIGURE 5-16—*Comparison of normal blood flow in a ten-year-old boy with intact ventricular septum (upper panel) to a patient with two muscular ventricular defects (lower panel) with systolic gating (small arrows on ECG). The upper panel depicts an apical four-chamber view of a normal heart. The flow stream along the left side of the interventricular septum is normal. In the modified subcostal four-chamber view (lower panel) there are two blue jets (open arrows) arising from the left ventricle into the right ventricle, indicating two apical defects. LV = left ventricle; RV = right ventricle.* (Reproduced with permission from Ludomirsky A, Huhta JC, Vick GW, et al: Color Doppler detection of multiple ventricular septal defects. Circulation 74:1317-1322, 1986.)

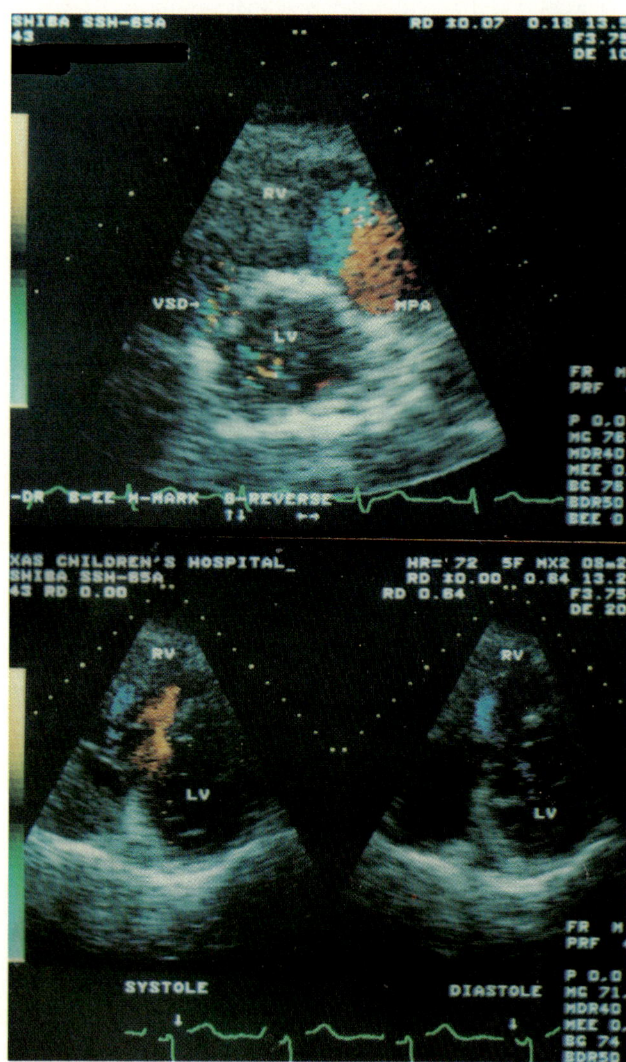

FIGURE 5-17—*Large ventricular septal defect in a two-year-old girl shows color Doppler of flow entering the large pulmonary artery depicted in blue away from the transducer (upper panel). A large shunt causes increased blood flow in the main pulmonary artery and aliasing (red-orange color). The lower panel shows a 33-year-old patient with ventricular septal defect and pulmonary hypertension and bidirectional shunting (red in systole and blue in diastole). LA = left atrium; MPA = main pulmonary artery; VSD = ventricular septal defect.*

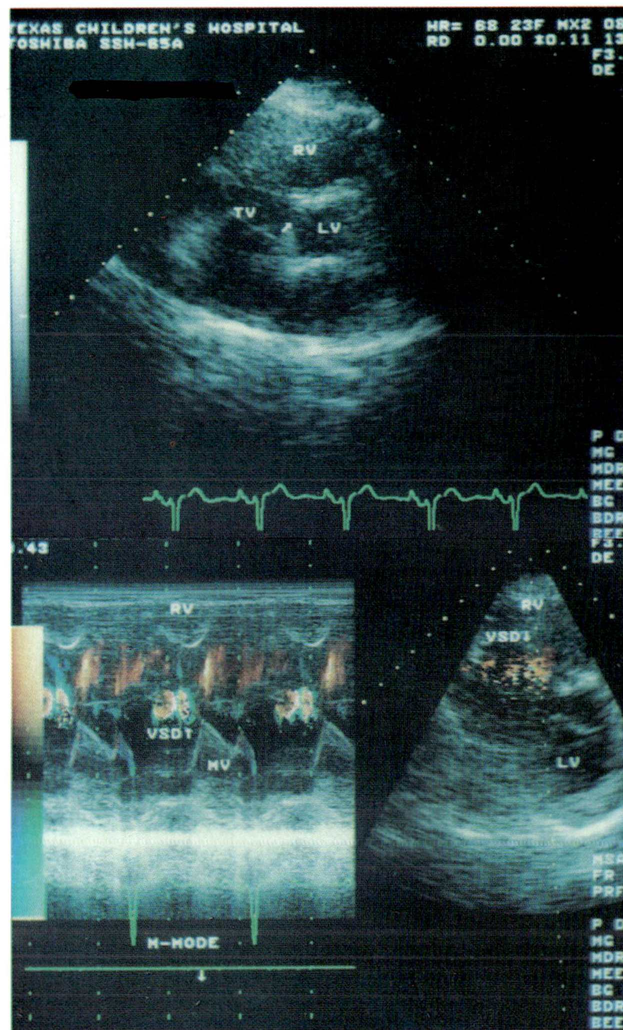

FIGURE 5-18—*M-mode color in ventricular septal defect showing VSD shunt with variance in systole in a perimembranous defect. LV = left ventricle; MV = mitral valve; RV = right ventricle; VSD = ventricle septal defect; TV = tricuspid valve.*

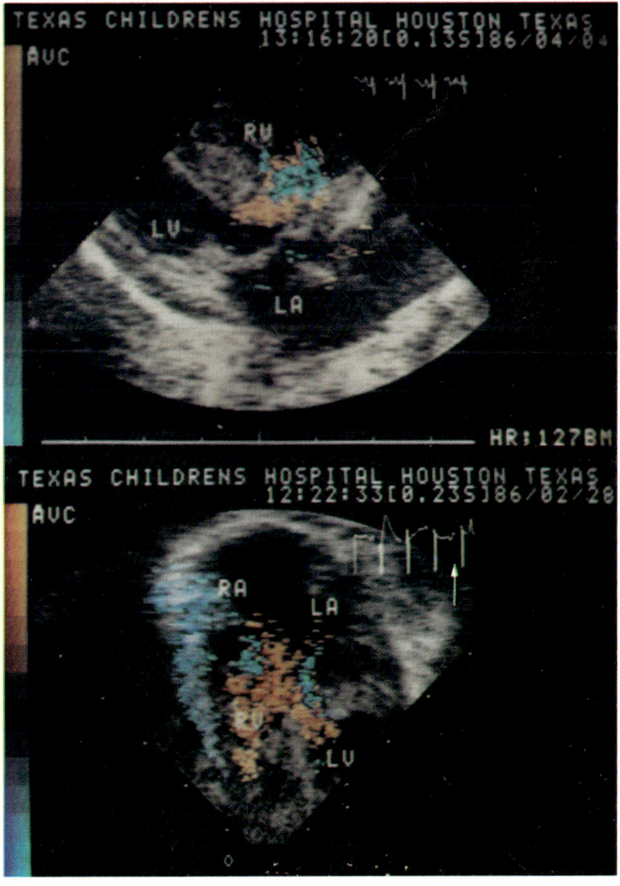

FIGURE 5-19—*Complete atrioventricular canal defect (AVC) with color Doppler. In the parasternal long-axis view, the typical AVC defect with a large shunt shows a systolic jet with variance from the left ventricle to the right ventricle during systole (upper panel). The apical four-chamber view in another patient reveals simultaneous filling of both ventricles in diastole (lower panel). Abbreviations as above.*

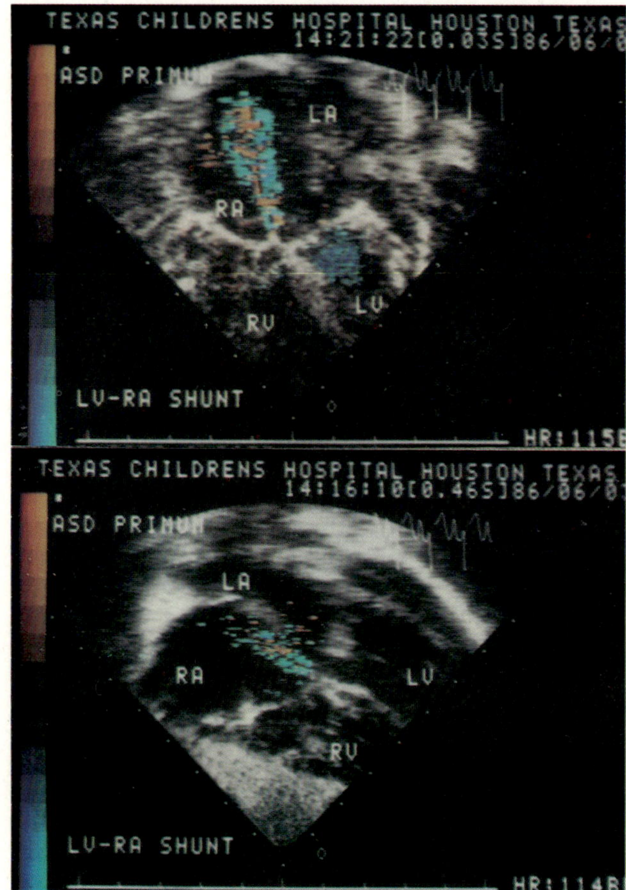

FIGURE 5-20—*Partial form of atrioventricular septal defect (primum ASD) with left ventricular to right atrial shunt jet. The detection of left ventricular to right atrial shunt is one of the advantages of color Doppler in this lesion for the differentiation from interventricular shunting and tricuspid regurgitation (see Figure 5-22). The detection of the LV-RA jet is possible with apical (upper panel) and subcostal (lower panel) views. LA = left atrium; LV = left ventricle; RA = right atrium; RV = right ventricle.*

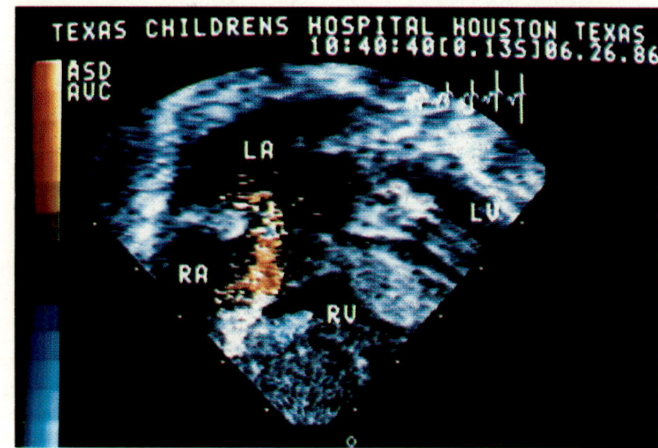

FIGURE 5-21—*Subcostal view of a left atrial (LA) to right atrial (RA) shunt in a partial AVC defect. Aliasing is present owing to the large volume of shunt at a relatively high velocity. Abbreviations as above.*

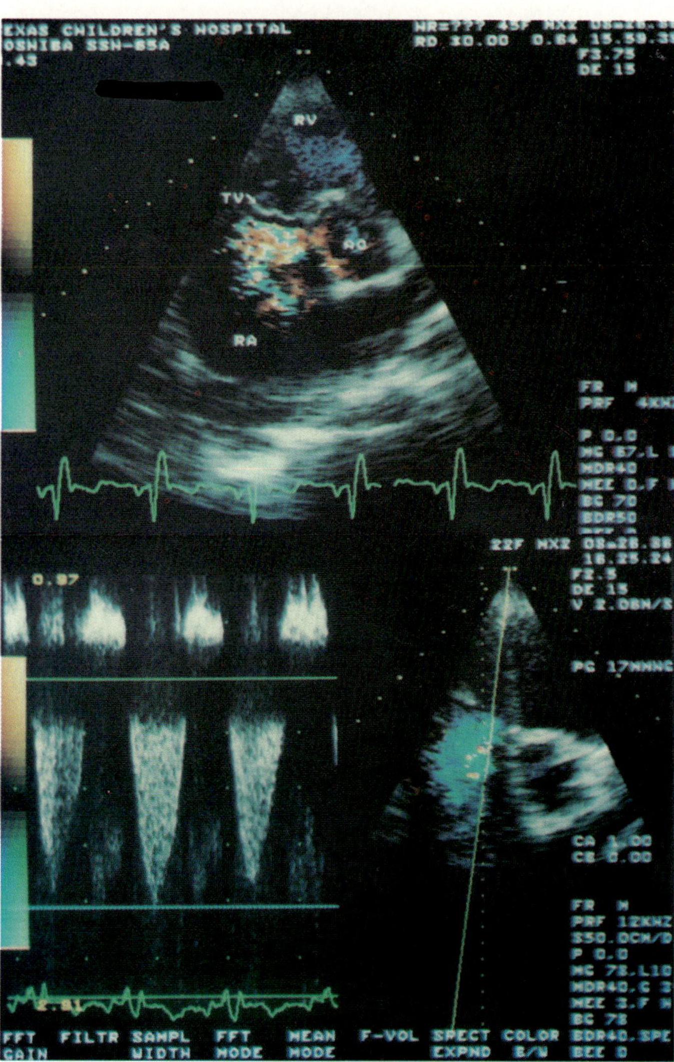

FIGURE 5-22—*Detection and quantitation of tricuspid regurgitation in a patient with a partial AVC defect (ostium primum ASD). Continuous-wave Doppler showed a peak velocity of 2 meters per second, compatible with normal right ventricular pressure. Note the variance in the shunt (upper panel) compared to the pattern in the tricuspid insufficiency jet (lower panel). AO = aorta; RA = right atrium; RV = right ventricle; TV = tricuspid valve.*

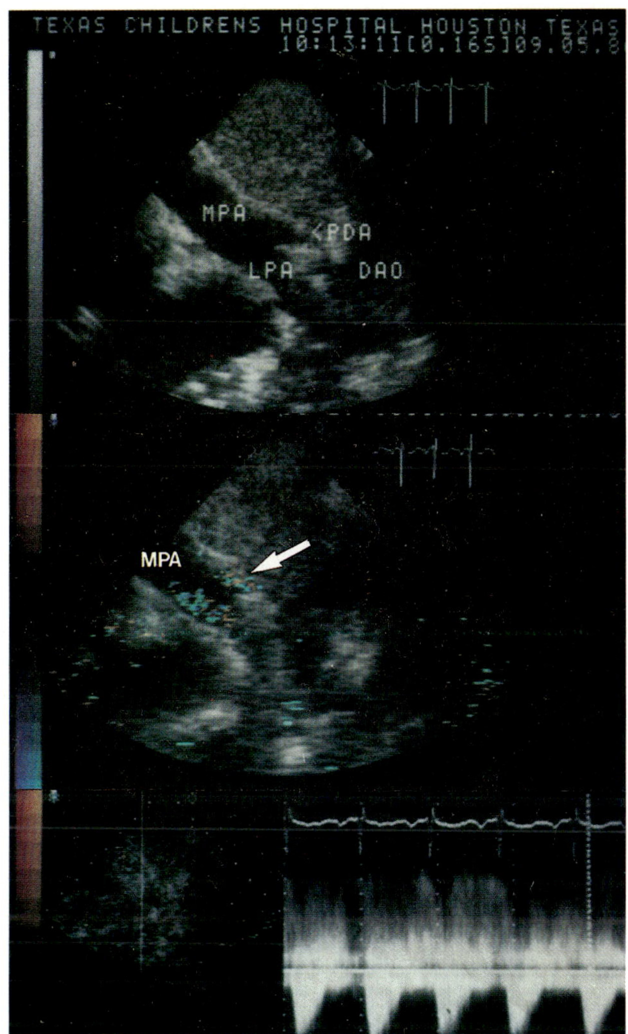

FIGURE 5-23—*Patent ductus arteriosus (PDA) measuring 3 millimeters in diameter and detected by color Doppler (middle panel). The peak gradient across the PDA by continuous-wave Doppler is 50 mmHg (3.5 meters per second jet [lower panel]). DAO = descending aorta; LPA = left pulmonary artery; MPA = main pulmonary artery.*

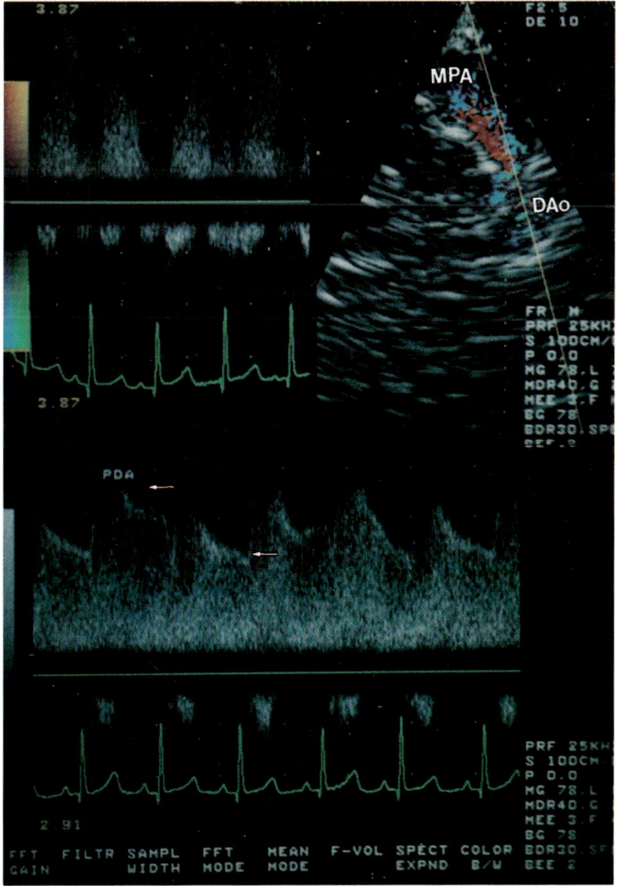

FIGURE 5-24—*Color Doppler-directed continuous-wave Doppler of a patent ductus arteriosus (PDA). The sample line is placed between the main pulmonary artery and the descending aorta (DAo) (upper panel) and the maximum and minimum velocities of the jet (white arrows in the lower panel) indicate the ductal pressure gradients in systole and diastole.*

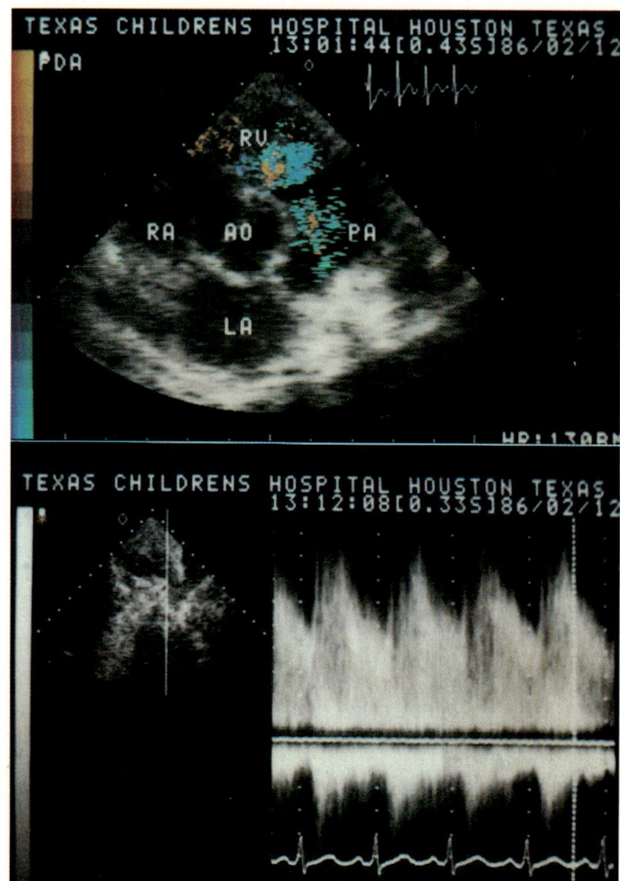

FIGURE 5-25—*Color Doppler sampling similar to Figure 5-24 in a patient with PDA with a large aorta to pulmonary artery pressure gradient. AO = aortic valve; LA = left atrium; PA = pulmonary artery; RA = right atrium; RV = right ventricle.*

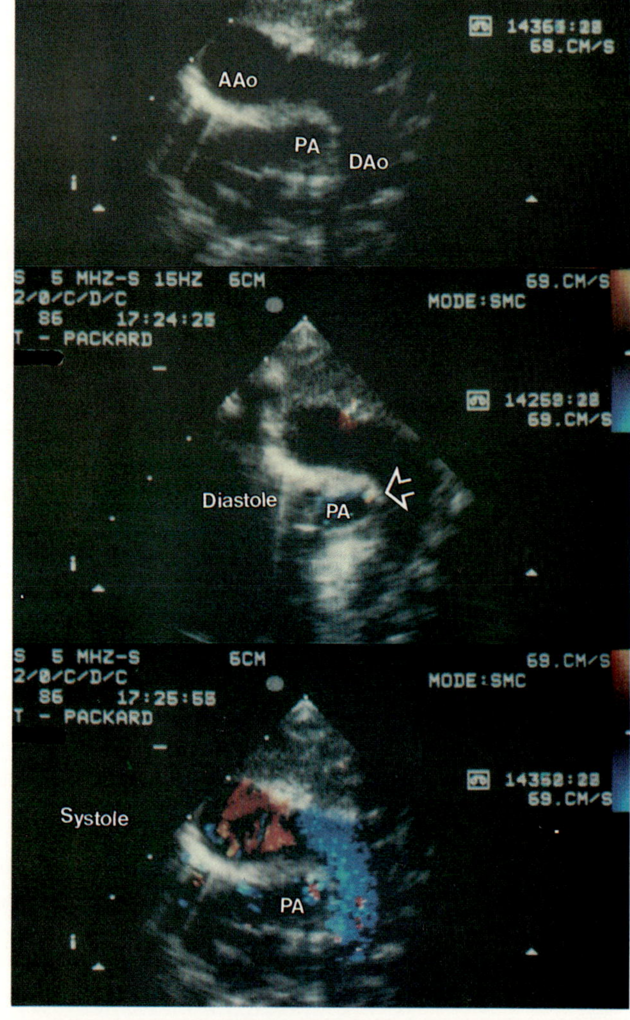

FIGURE 5-26—*Color Doppler of the aortic arch from a high parasternal approach showing a diastolic frame with continuous flow in a small ductus under the aortic arch (open arrow in the middle panel), and a systolic frame with large aortic flow and aliasing and variance of the color Doppler display (lower panel). AAo = ascending aorta; DAo = descending aorta; PA = pulmonary artery.*

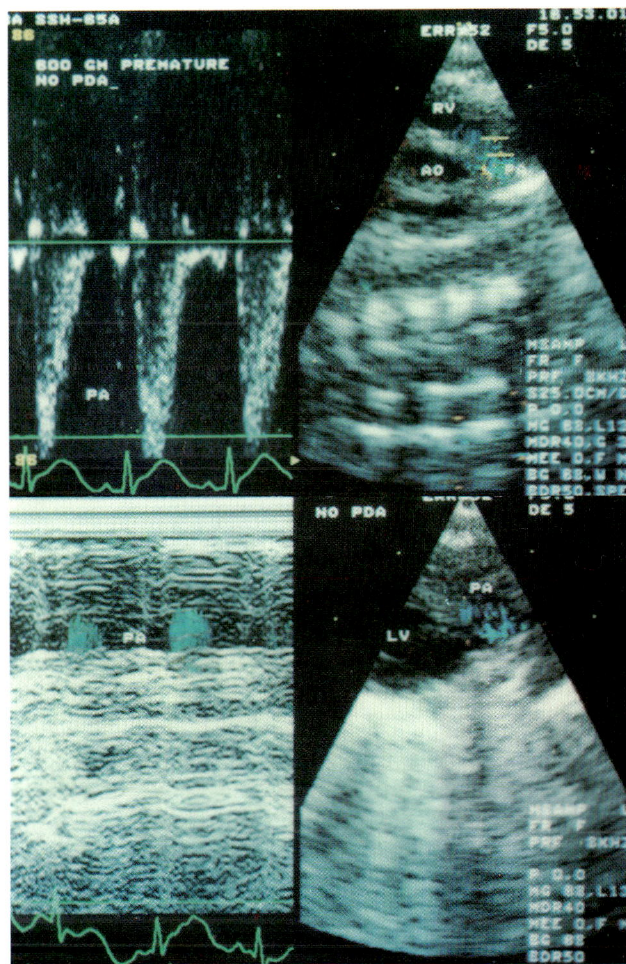

FIGURE 5-27—*Pulsed Doppler and color Doppler in a 600 gram premature infant. The systolic velocity of 0.9 meters per second is normal and there is no evidence of a diastolic abnormality typical of a PDA either by pulsed (upper panel) or color/M-mode Doppler (lower panel).*

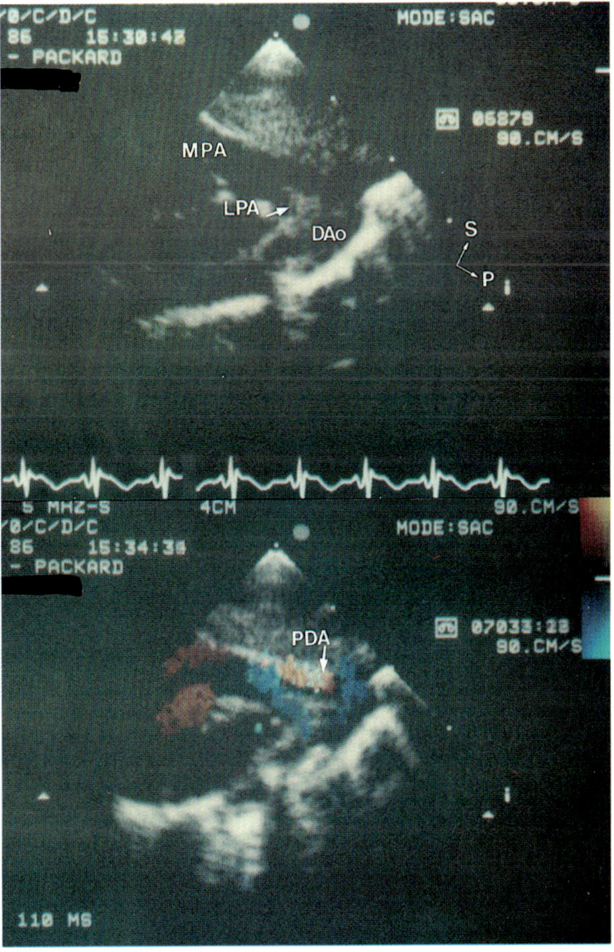

FIGURE 5-28—*High parasternal scan of a premature infant in search of a patent ductus arteriosus (PDA). Imaging of the main pulmonary artery (MPA) and descending aorta (DAo) is equivocal (upper panel) but color Doppler readily shows a prominent diastolic jet of PDA (lower panel). LPA = left pulmonary artery.*

References

1. Tajik AJ, Seward JB, Hagler DJ, et al: Two-dimensional real-time ultrasonic imaging of the heart and great vessels: Technique, image orientation, structure identification and validation. Mayo Clin Proc 53:271-303, 1978.
2. Hatle L, Angelsen B: Doppler Ultrasound in Cardiology—Physical Principles and Clinical Applications, 2nd ed. Philadelphia, Lea & Febiger, 1985.
3. Stevenson JG, Kawabori I, Stamm SJ, et al: Pulsed Doppler echocardiographic evaluation of ventricular septal defect patches. Circulation 70(Suppl I):38-46, 1984.
4. Stevenson JG: Multigated Doppler visualization of intracardiac flow disturbances in congenital heart disease. In Spencer MP (ed): Cardiac Doppler Diagnosis. Boston, Martinus Nijhoff, 1983, p 235.
5. Shub C, Dimopoulos IN, Seward JB, et al: Sensitivity of two-dimensional echocardiography in the direct visualization of atrial septal defect utilizing the subcostal approach: Experience with 154 patients. J Am Coll Cardiol 2(1):127, 135, 1982.
6. Suzuki Y, Kambara H, Kadota K, et al: Detection of intracardiac shunt flow in atrial septal defect using a real-time two-dimensional color-coded Doppler flow imaging system and comparison with contrast two-dimensional echocardiography. Am J Cardiol 56:347-350, 1985.
7. Murphy DJ, Ludomirsky A, Huhta JC: Continuous wave Doppler in children with ventricular septal defect: Noninvasive estimation of interventricular pressure gradient. Am J Cardiol 57:428-432, 1986.
8. Valdes-Cruz LM, Horowitz S, Mesel E, et al: A pulsed Doppler echocardiographic method for calculating pulmonary and systemic blood flow in atrial level shunts: Validation studies in animals and initial human experience. Circulation 69:80-86, 1984.
9. Valdes-Cruz LM, Horowitz S, Mesel E, et al: A pulsed Doppler echocardiographic method for calculation of pulmonary and systemic flow: Accuracy in a canine model with ventricular septal defect. Circulation 68:597, 1983.
10. Ortiz E, Robinson PJ, Dearfield JE, et al: Localization of ventricular septal defects by simultaneous display of superimposed colour Doppler and cross sectional echocardiographic images. Br Heart J 54:53-60, 1985.
11. Ludomirsky A, Huhta JC, Vick GW, et al: Color Doppler detection of multiple ventricular septal defects. Circulation 74, 1317-1322, 1986.
12. Hagler DJ, Mair DD, Tajik AJ, et al: Real-time wide-angle sector echocardiography: Atrioventricular canal defects. Circulation 59:140-149, 1979.
13. Smallhorn JF, Tommasini G, Anderson RH, et al: Assessment of atrioventricular septal defects by two-dimensional echocardiography. Br Heart J 47:109-121, 1982.
14. Colvin E, Nanda N, Bargeron LM: Color Doppler flow mapping in atrioventricular septal defects. Circulation 72(Suppl III):III-436, 1985 (abstr).
15. Vick GW, Huhta JC, Gutgesell HP: Assessment of the ductus arteriosus in preterm infants utilizing suprasternal two-dimensional/Doppler echocardiography. J Am Coll Cardiol 5:973-977, 1985.

Chapter 6

Complex Congenital Heart Disease

Daniel J. Murphy Jr., M.D., and James C. Huhta, M.D.

The presence of complex congenital heart disease usually means that there is cyanosis which is due to one or more factors: (1) right-to-left shunting with reduced pulmonary blood flow, (2) complete intracardiac mixing with or without pulmonary edema, (3) differential streaming of desaturated blood to the body despite increased pulmonary blood flow, or (4) impaired pulmonary function due to pulmonary edema. Doppler echocardiography in general and color Doppler in particular assists the clinician in determining the sites and patterns of blood flow.[1,2] In this chapter each lesion is discussed separately and the characteristic color flow patterns are described and illustrated.

Tetralogy of Fallot

The major hemodynamic components of tetralogy of Fallot are a ventricular septal defect and infundibular and valvular pulmonary stenosis. In general, peak right and left ventricular pressures are equal. In "pink" tetralogy, the net flow across the ventricular septal defect is from left to right although there is always bidirectional shunting. As the pulmonary stenosis becomes more severe, cyanosis develops and net flow across the ventricular septal defect (VSD) occurs from right to left. Systolic flow from both ventricles enters the ascending aorta with significant right-to-left shunting. The direction of VSD flow is easily demonstrated using color Doppler and provides corroborative information regarding the resistance to pulmonary flow (Figure 6-1).

Patients with tetralogy of Fallot may have either infundibular and valvular pulmonary stenosis or pulmonary atresia. The typical color flow pattern demonstrates high-velocity (aliasing) systolic flow in the pulmonary artery. In the absence of significant collateral flow or patent ductus arteriosus, no diastolic flow should be demonstrable in the main pulmonary artery.

Electrocardiographic gating in diastole should detect the presence of retrograde diastolic flow due to a patent ductus. In the patient with pulmonary atresia, color flow mapping reveals continuous flow but no posteriorly directed systolic flow in the main pulmonary artery. Because of the small size of the main pulmonary artery in such patients, color flow mapping provides a distinct advantage over routine pulsed Doppler examination in which the sample volume must be placed precisely in the main pulmonary artery.

Tetralogy of Fallot is frequently accompanied by peripheral stenosis of the pulmonary arteries. This occurs at or near the bifurcation of the main pulmonary artery. Such branch stenosis is poorly demonstrated by color Doppler owing to upstream flow disturbance and acceleration at the level of the infundibular and pulmonary valve. Tricuspid regurgitation is commonly present in patients with tetralogy of Fallot postoperatively and is easily demonstrated using color flow mapping (see the discussion of postoperative tetralogy in Chapter 8). Finally, a careful, complete color Doppler examination will exclude or detect the presence of any unexpected associated flow abnormalities such as aortic insufficiency or atrial septal defect.

Transposition of the Great Arteries

In complete transposition of the great arteries (d-transposition), intracardiac flow patterns are essentially normal, with the exception of mixing at the level of the atrial septal defect. Color Doppler is used to confirm the presence of bidirectional flow and to assess the flow area (size of atrial defect). Studies before and after balloon atrial septostomy demonstrate the usefulness of this technique in confirming the improvement in intracardiac mixing. In addition, increased velocities across a restrictive atrial septal defect can be detected using color flow mapping techniques.

The detection of *left ventricular outflow tract obstruction* or valvular pulmonic stenosis can be facilitated using color flow mapping. In addition to para-

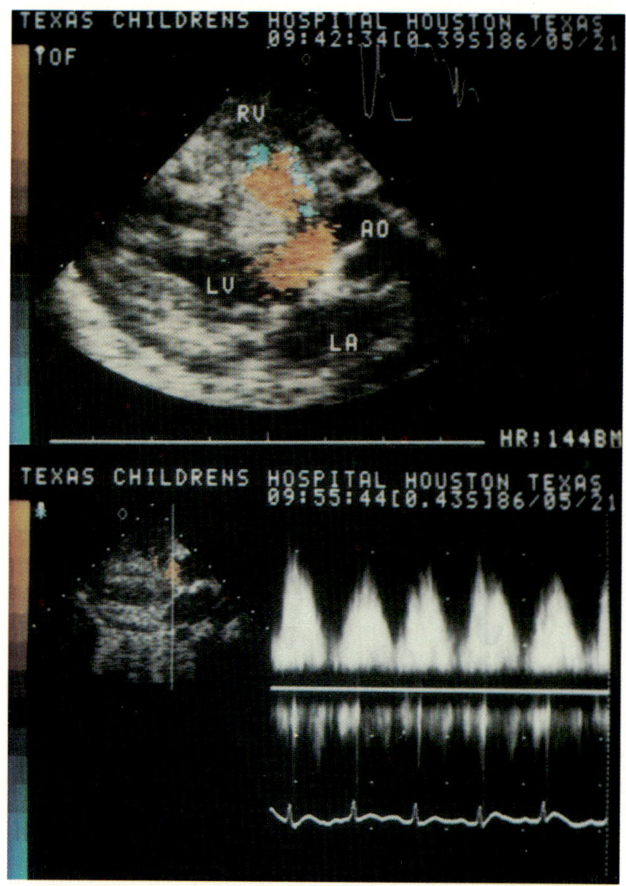

FIGURE 6-1—*Tetralogy of Fallot with typical overriding aorta (Ao) and ventricular septal defect between the left (LV) and right ventricles (RV). A systolic frame shows left-to-right shunting by color Doppler. Continuous-wave Doppler confirms left-to-right shunt in (lower panel). LA = left atrium.*

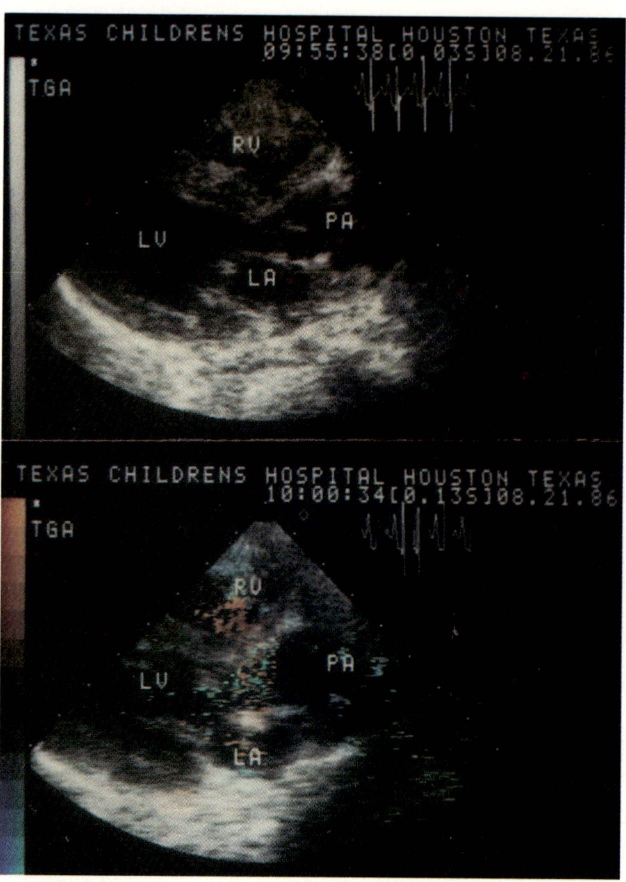

FIGURE 6-2—*Color Doppler in transposition of the great arteries (TGA) with intact ventricular septum and no left ventricular outflow tract obstruction between the left ventricle (LV) and the pulmonary artery (PA). There is aliasing in the proximal PA which may occur without significant obstruction. RV = right ventricle; LA = left atrium.*

sternal scans showing the usual mitral-pulmonary valve continuity (Figure 6-2), color Doppler can be used to examine for abnormal turbulence in the pulmonary artery. Swirling of blood due to valvular or subvalvular pulmonary stenosis may be difficult to differentiate from the continuous flow disturbance that is produced by the presence of a patent ductus arteriosus. From the high parasternal window, a PDA produces diastolic flow toward the transducer in the main pulmonary artery (see Chapter 5).

In transposition of the great arteries with ventricular septal defect (Figure 6-3), the direction of flow across the VSD is determined by the relative ventricular pressures. In the absence of left ventricular outflow tract obstruction, flow primarily occurs from the right ventricle to the left. On color Doppler this flow is seen occurring in systole away from the transducer in the parasternal views. The stream of blood across the ventricular defect mixes with the blood already in the left ventricular outflow tract to produce one pattern of flow disturbance in the left ventricular outflow tract. The presence of left ventricular hypertension causes bidirectional shunting across the ventricular septum and a systolic jet oriented toward the transducer can be identified. Color Doppler is of most benefit in situations where there are two abnormal jets intermixing, such as those from a VSD and subpulmonary stenosis in transposition of the great arteries.

For patients with transposition in whom atrial switch procedures (Mustard or Senning) are contemplated, the presence of tricuspid regurgitation is clinically important (see Chapter 8). From the parasternal short-axis and the modified apical views, tricuspid regurgitation can be detected and its severity estimated.

Pulmonary Atresia

In patients with *pulmonary atresia and intact ventricular septum*, the right ventricle is hypoplastic, as

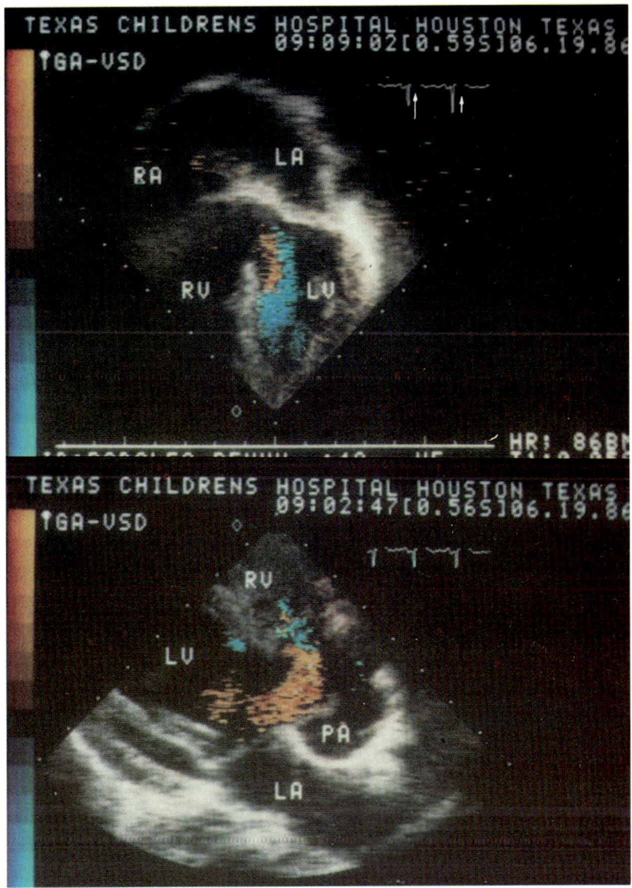

FIGURE 6-3—*Transposition of the great arteries with a large ventricular septal defect (TGA-VSD). The apical scan shows aliasing at the defect on a frame gated in systole (white arrows on ECG). There is overriding of the pulmonary artery (PA) and systolic shunt from the left (LV) to right (RV) ventricle (lower panel). LA = left atrium; RA = right atrium.*

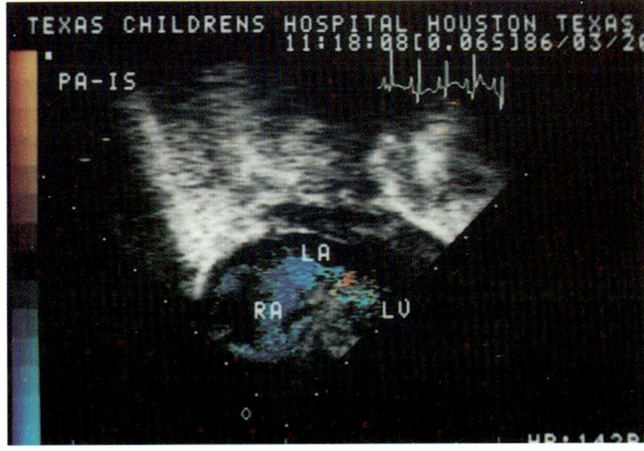

FIGURE 6-4—*Right-to-left atrial shunting in pulmonary atresia with intact ventricular septum (PA-IS). LA = left atrium; LV = left ventricle; RA = right atrium.*

is the tricuspid valve annulus and apparatus. Typically, flow into the right ventricle through the tricuspid valve is of low velocity and small volume, and therefore frequently is not detected by using color flow mapping. However, the blood that does enter the right ventricle is often ejected from the ventricle through an insufficient tricuspid valve. This tricuspid insufficiency can be detected using color Doppler (Figure 6-4) and the peak velocity can be used to predict the right ventricular pressure.

In pulmonary atresia with intact septum, the entire systemic and pulmonary output must cross the atrial septal defect. As in patients with transposition of the great arteries, the atrial septal defect flow area can be estimated and the results of balloon atrial septostomy can be assessed by color Doppler (Figure 6-4).

Pulmonary artery flow in pulmonary atresia occurs throughout systole and diastole but its pulsatile character can make it difficult to separate from antegrade pulmonary valve flow when there is a widely patent ductus arteriosus. Color Doppler is extremely useful in detecting the presence of antegrade pulmonary valve flow which may be confused with a late systolic jet through the ductus arteriosus. This is essential to know if pulmonary valvuloplasty is being considered as a method of treatment in the catheterization laboratory. Surveillence of the state of the ductus is possible with color Doppler (see Chapter 5) and is important because the patient's clinical status is dependent on ductal patency which is necessary for survival prior to surgical intervention.

Because the entire systemic and pulmonary output crosses the mitral and aortic valves, the flow velocities across these structures are increased. The increased flow velocities are demonstrated by color Doppler as aliasing of the color flow signal (Figure 6-5). This pattern is not due to structural stenosis of the valves involved; rather, it represents a functional restriction of flow due to increased flow volume and the velocities rarely exceed 1.6 to 1.8 meters per second.

Tricuspid Atresia

A broad spectrum of anatomical abnormalities exist in patients with the clinical diagnosis of tricuspid atresia. Intracardiac communications at the atrial and ventricular levels are essential for survival. Color flow mapping can be used to demonstrate these communications and qualitatively estimate the flow areas (Figure 6-6). Color flow jets can be used to guide pulsed and continuous-wave Doppler studies for the purpose of detecting maximal systolic velocities. Pulmonary stenosis—both subvalvular and valvular—is common in patients

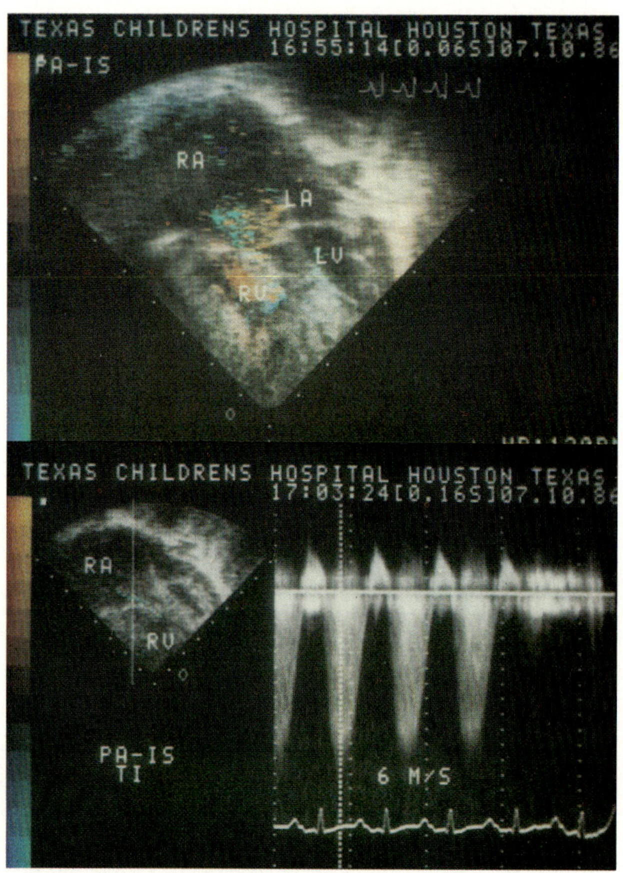

FIGURE 6-5—*Color and continuous-wave Doppler in an infant with pulmonary atresia and intact ventricular septum (PA-IS) with tricuspid insufficiency (TI) with a peak velocity of 6 meters per second which correctly predicted a right ventricular (RV) pressure of greater than 150 mmHg. LA = left atrium; LV = left ventricle; RA = right atrium.*

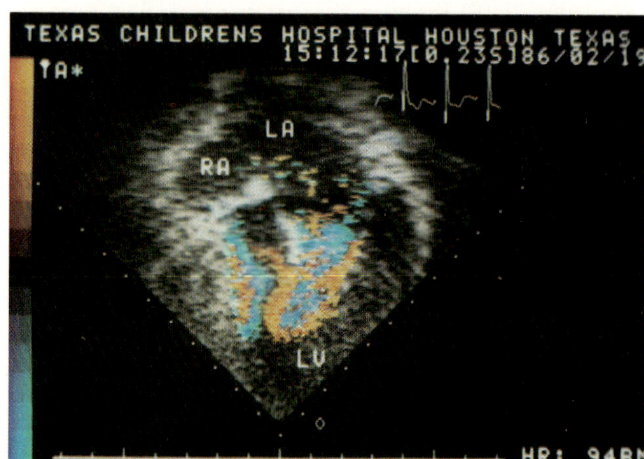

FIGURE 6-6—*Interatrial shunting from the right atrium (RA) to the left atrium (LA) in an adolescent with tricuspid atresia (TA). Note the diastolic left ventricular (LV) filling velocity pattern on color Doppler.*

with tricuspid atresia, and proper transducer location allows one to detect the resultant flow disturbance. Many patients with tricuspid atresia have subpulmonary obstruction at the ventricular septal defect. With normally related great arteries, parasternal continuous-wave Doppler can be used to measure the VSD gradient (Figure 6-7). Because both the systemic and pulmonary circulations traverse the mitral valve, there is a relative increase in flow velocity which can be detected with color Doppler. Mitral valve function is crucial to a successful surgical result using the modified Fontan approach and mitral valve insufficiency can be detected with ease from apical or parasternal long-axis scans.

Truncus Arteriosus

In truncus arteriosus there is a large subarterial ventricular septal defect and the pulmonary arteries arise from the ascending aorta. The ventricular septal defect is rarely restrictive and there is no pulmonary valve. The parasternal long-axis image appears similar to that of pulmonary atresia with VSD or tetralogy. Systolic truncal valve flow is high; however, the truncal valve may be stenotic and truncal valve insufficiency is common (Figure 6-8). Color flow examination of the patient with truncus arteriosus should include careful examination of the flow patterns in the ascending aorta. Detection of truncal stenosis, however, can be difficult because flow volume across the truncal valve is increased as well as blood flow velocity. When truncal valve stenosis is suspected, careful pulsed and continuous-wave Doppler studies should be performed to document the flow disturbance and to quantitate the peak systolic velocities. It is clinically important to detect and quantify truncal insufficiency during the echocardiographic examination. The techniques in truncus arteriosus are similar to those used for quantitation of aortic insufficiency (see Chapter 4). As with pulmonary atresia- VSD, valve insufficiency can produce a diastolic jet into the right ventricle and this is better appreciated with color Doppler than with pulsed or continuous-wave techniques (Figure 6-9).

Double Outlet Right Ventricle

Patients with doublet outlet right ventricle depend on the presence of a large ventricular septal defect for survival. The ventricular septal defect can be imaged using two-dimensional echocardiography and the flow patterns across it examined using color flow mapping.

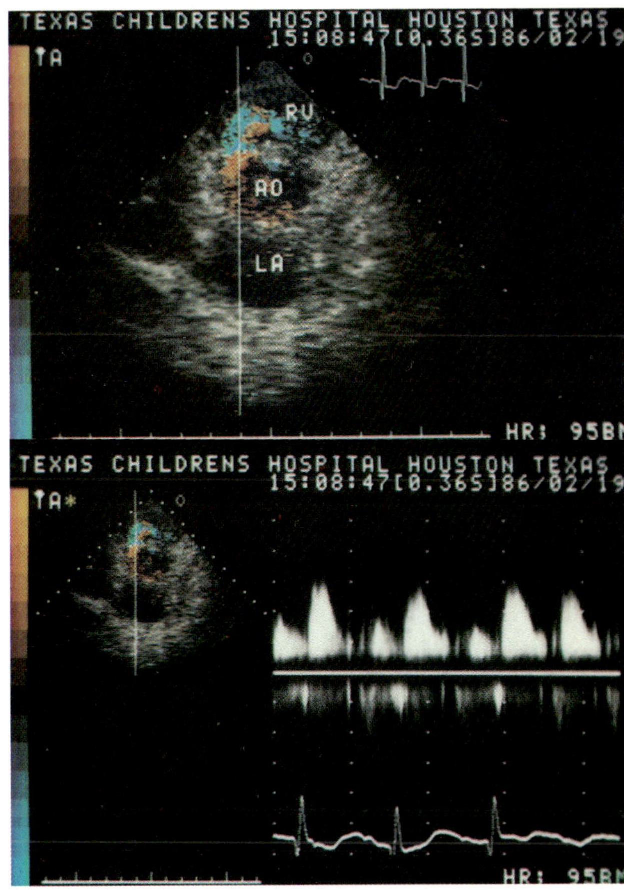

FIGURE 6-7—*Assessment of the ventricular septal defect in tricuspid atresia and normally related great arteries. There is no significant obstruction at this level and the velocity is only 1 meter per second. AO = aorta; LA = left atrium; RV = right ventricle.*

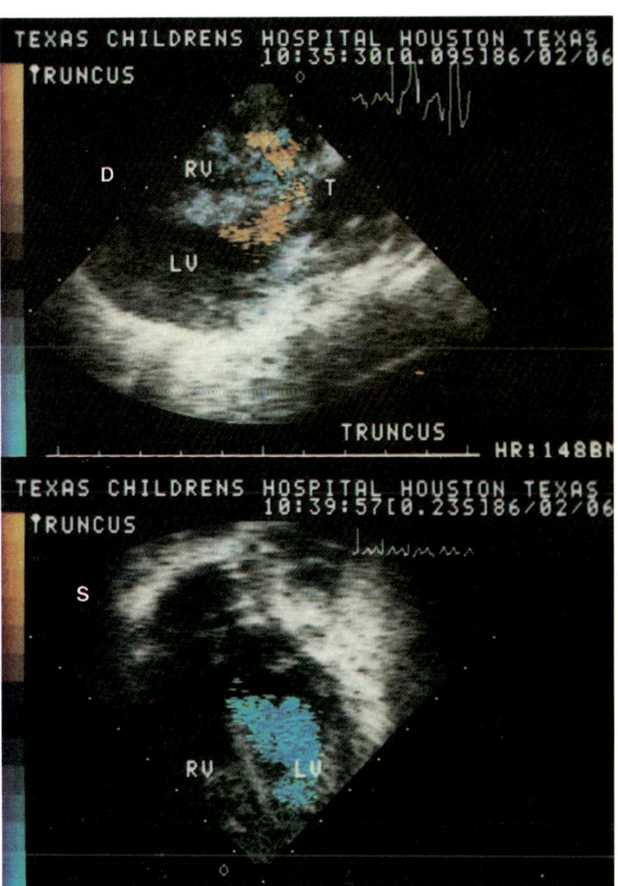

FIGURE 6-8—*Truncal valve (T) insufficiency into both left (LV) and right (RV) ventricles on a parasternal scan. An apical view shows variance at the VSD in systole (lower panel). D = diastole; S = systole.*

Systolic and sometimes diastolic shunting occur at this level depending on the magnitude of pulmonary blood flow. Restrictive VSD should produce increased velocities and the pattern should guide the performance of a continuous-wave examination for determination of peak systolic velocity. An important point for the clinician is the assessment of the amount of pulmonary blood flow that returns to the pulmonary artery that is "trapped" in the left heart if there is no atrial septal defect.

Obstruction to aortic and/or pulmonary flow can occur in patients with double outlet right ventricle. Therefore, the flow patterns in the aorta and main pulmonary arteries should be examined carefully in such patients.

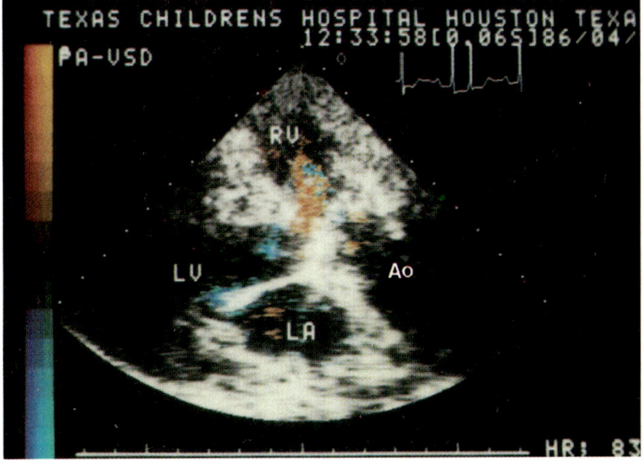

FIGURE 6-9—*Aortic valve insufficiency into the right ventricle in pulmonary atresia with ventricular septal defect (PA-VSD) on a diastolic frame. Ao = aorta; LA = left atrium; LV = left ventricle; RV = right ventricle.*

Hypoplastic Left Heart Syndrome

The most striking abnormal flow pattern in hypoplastic left heart syndrome is that of systolic retrograde flow in the ascending aorta and aortic valve due to aortic atresia. Color Doppler reveals flow directed toward the transducer from the suprasternal notch in the proximal descending aorta and flow directed away from the transducer in the ascending aorta. Newborn infants with hypoplastic left heart syndrome require an atrial septal defect and patent ductus arteriosus for survival. Flow across the atrial septum can be imaged with color Doppler and a restrictive atrial septal defect produces high-velocity flows with a different characteristic than flow across a large ASD. Flow across the patent ductus arteriosus occurs primarily right to left during systole; however, there may be some low-velocity left-to-right flow. Tricuspid regurgitation (see Chapter 4) occurs commonly in infants with hypoplastic left heart syndrome. In fact, survival may be related to the degree of tricuspid regurgitation and color Doppler provides an estimate of the amount of regurgitant flow.

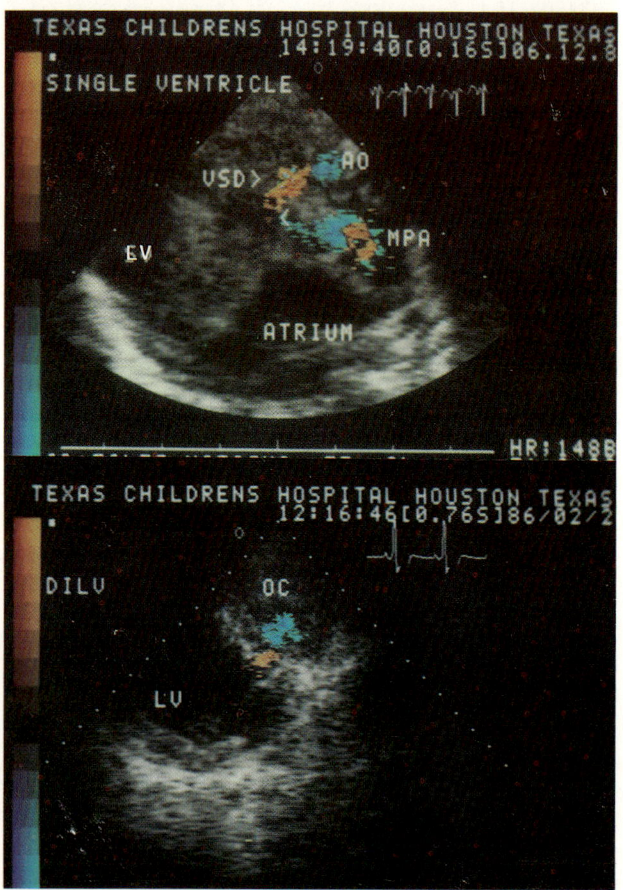

FIGURE 6-10—*Two patients with double inlet ventricle and transposition with mild obstruction of the ventricular septal defect between the left ventricle (LV) and the RV outlet chamber (OC). The main pulmonary artery (MPA) is posterior with a narrow jet with aliasing and variance compatible with pulmonary stenosis (upper panel).*

Double Inlet Ventricle (Single Ventricle)

There is a broad spectrum of complex congenital abnormalities that include a univentricular atrioventricular connection, that is, to one ventricle—either double inlet or common inlet.[3] Patients with single inlet (tricuspid atresia or mitral atresia) have similar hemodynamics and associated anomalies. Double inlet to the left ventricle means two atrioventricular valves draining to the main ventricular chamber. The presence of obstruction of either valve is of great clinical importance and this has led to wide application of Doppler in this situation. This is most important if there is severe pulmonary stenosis or atresia and if a surgical shunt to increase pulmonary blood flow is being considered. If the left atrioventricular valve is stenotic, then an atrial septal defect must be created.

The connection of the great arteries (normal connection or transposition) greatly affects the clinical impact of the malformation. With transposition, the blood flow to the body must pass through the ventricular septal defect, which may be restrictive, thereby causing subaortic stenosis between the left ventricle and the right ventricular outlet chamber (Figure 6-10). In the presence of pulmonary stenosis, the main pulmonary artery will demonstrate poststenotic dilation (Figures 6-11 and 6-12). Common inlet with a common atrioventricular valve is usually part of the asplenia syndrome (see below).

Ebstein's Malformation

Ebstein's malformation is a complex disorder of the tricuspid valve with displacement of the leaflets into the right ventricular chamber causing "atrialization" of the right ventricle. This affects the inflow to the right ventricle which is reduced in size in proportion to the severity of the valve displacement. The atrialized right ventricle functions to restrict the flow of blood from the right atrium to the right ventricle and the valve leaflets are usually plastered down to the endocardium. Echocardiography is the mainstay of diagnostic techniques for Ebstein's.[4]

Color Doppler is useful in assessing the amount of blood exiting the right ventricle via the pulmonary valve. Tricuspid valve insufficiency occurs in this abnormality (Figure 6-13) but is not a common feature of the hemodynamic picture which is dominated by right-to-left shunting at the atrial level causing cyanosis. Newborn babies with Ebstein's can be difficult to evaluate by catheterization and careful Doppler examination using all modalities is extremely valuable before deciding on a treatment plan.

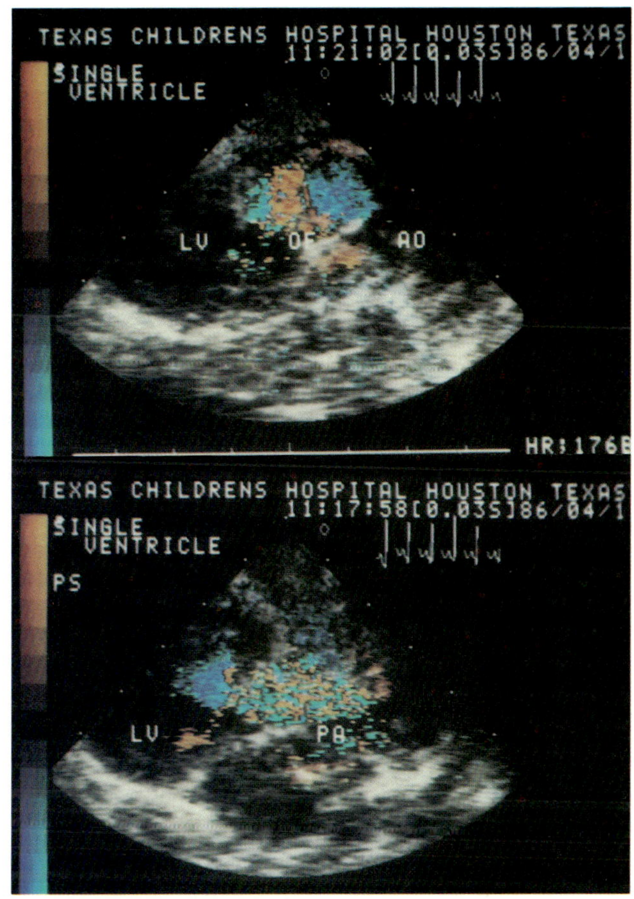

FIGURE 6-11—*Double inlet left ventricle (single ventricle) with no VSD obstruction but variance (upper panel) and pulmonary stenosis (lower panel) with poststenotic dilation. AO = aorta; LV = left ventricle; PA = pulmonary artery.*

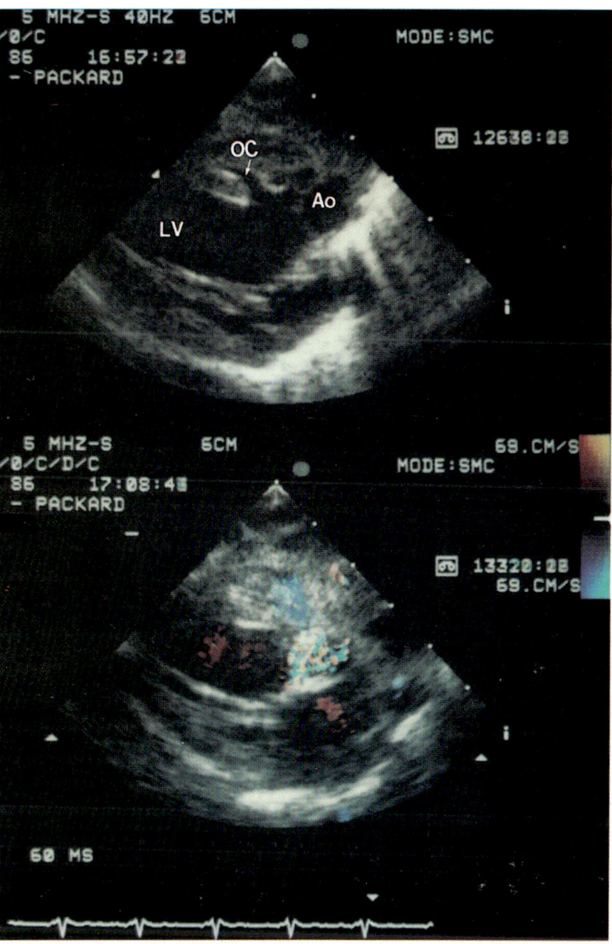

FIGURE 6-12—*Imaging and color Doppler in an infant with double inlet left ventricle (LV), a small RV outlet chamber (OC), and pulmonary stenosis (variance jet in lower panel color Doppler).*

Asplenia

Asplenia is common when there is abnormal atrial situs such that there are bilateral right atria (right atrial isomerism). Complex congenital heart disease is the rule with a combination of common inlet right ventricle (common atrioventricular valve), pulmonary valve stenosis or atresia, and total anomalous pulmonary venous connection, often with obstruction. The common valve may be regurgitant and this is a major factor in the prognosis. A combination of color and continuous-wave Doppler can exclude this problem (Figures 6-14 and 6-15). Identification of a left ventricular pouch may be aided by color Doppler if it communicates with the main right ventricular chamber (RV) (Figure 6-16). Color Doppler may be very important in identifying the presence of obstructed pulmonary venous return and the site of connection (Figure 6-17).

Corrected Transposition

In this abnormality there is atrioventricular discordance and ventriculoarterial discordance. The morphological right ventricle is the systemic ventricle and the tricuspid is often abnormal. Rarely, there is a form of Ebstein's malformation of this valve which can cause regurgitation (Figure 6-18) and is associated with a poor long-term survival.[5] There is an association with ventricular septal defect and pulmonary stenosis. If the stenosis is severe, systolic flow will be from the right-sided LV to the left-sided RV (Figure 6-19).

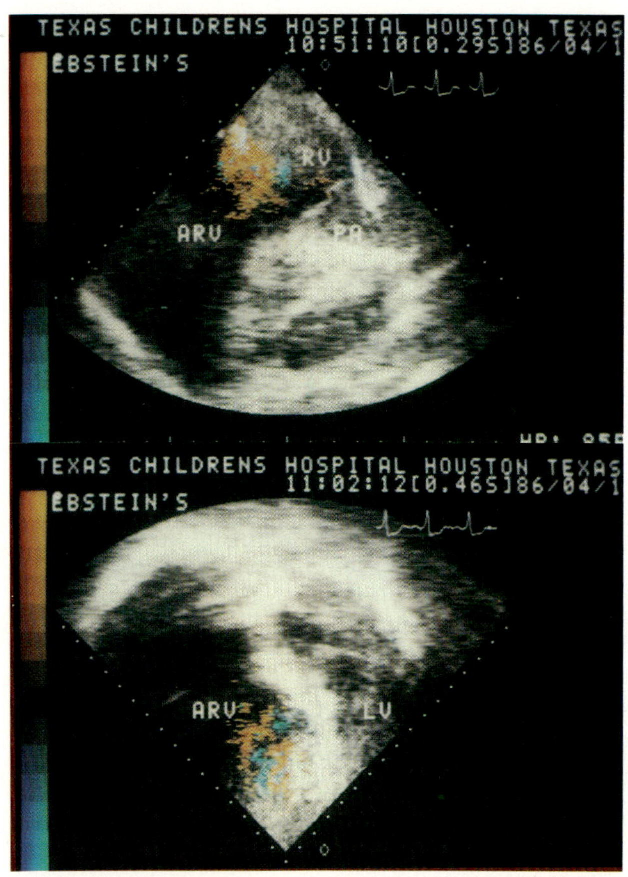

FIGURE 6-13—*Color Doppler in an adult with Ebstein's malformation of the tricuspid valve with valvular regurgitation into the atrialized right ventricle (ARV). LV* = left ventricle; PA = pulmonary artery; RV = true right ventricle.

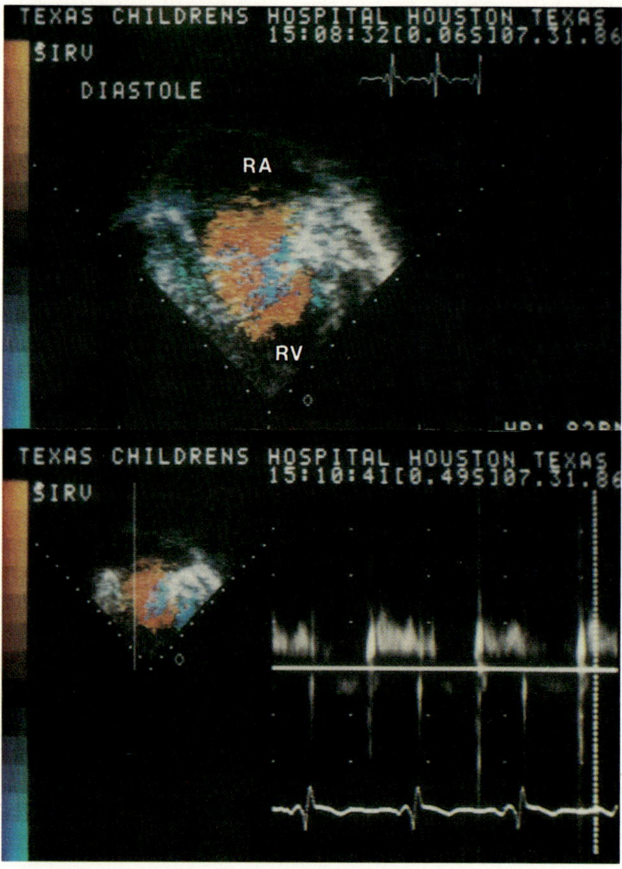

FIGURE 6-14—*Asplenia syndrome with a common inlet right ventricle (RV). Continuous-wave Doppler excludes any significant common AV valve insufficiency (lower panel). CA* = common atrium.

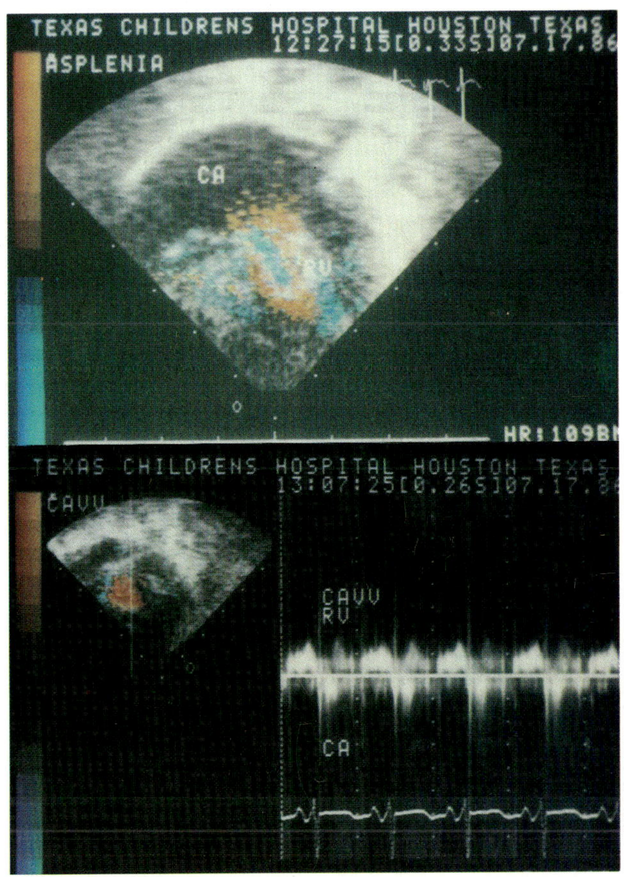

FIGURE 6-15—*Common inlet RV with mild common AV valve insufficiency on continuous-wave Doppler in a patient with asplenia syndrome. Color Doppler of diastole shows aliasing within the jet (upper panel). Abbreviations as in Figure 6-14.*

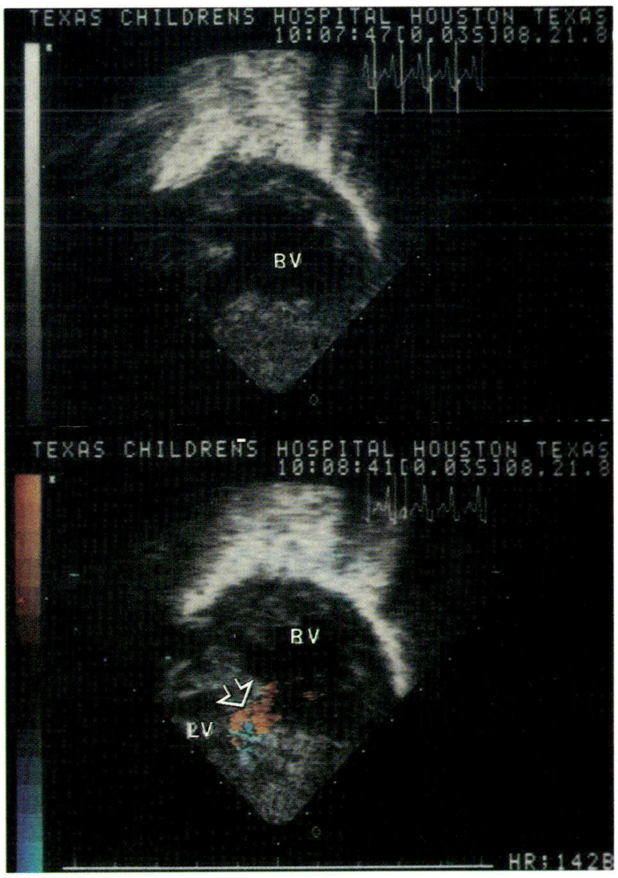

FIGURE 6-16—*Color Doppler identification (open white arrow) of communication between a small left ventricular pouch (LV) and the main right ventricular chamber (RV).*

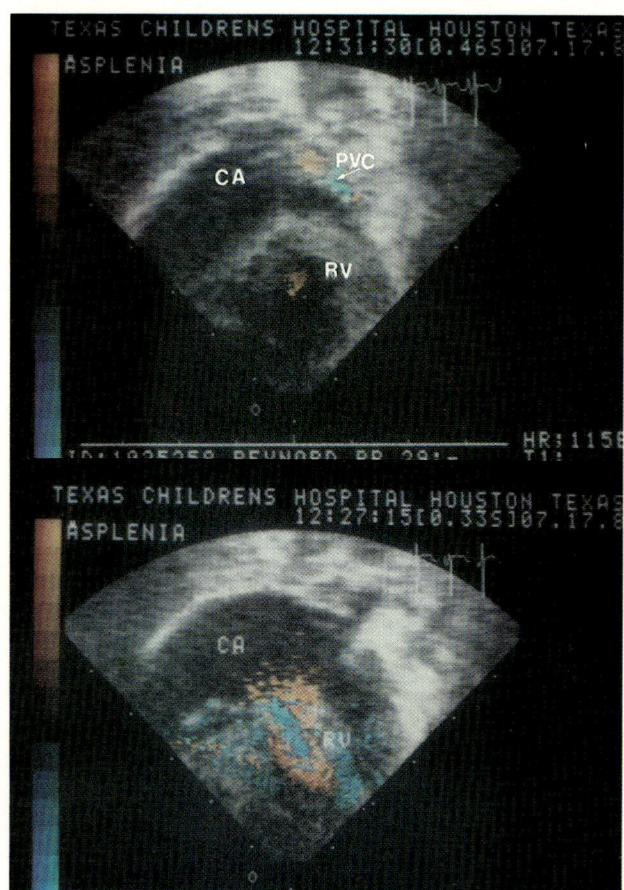

FIGURE 6-17—*Apical scans in an infant with pulmonary atresia and asplenia syndrome and total anomalous pulmonary venous connection. Color Doppler aids in the identification of the continuous flow in the pulmonary venous confluence (PVC). CA* = common atrium; RV = right ventricle.

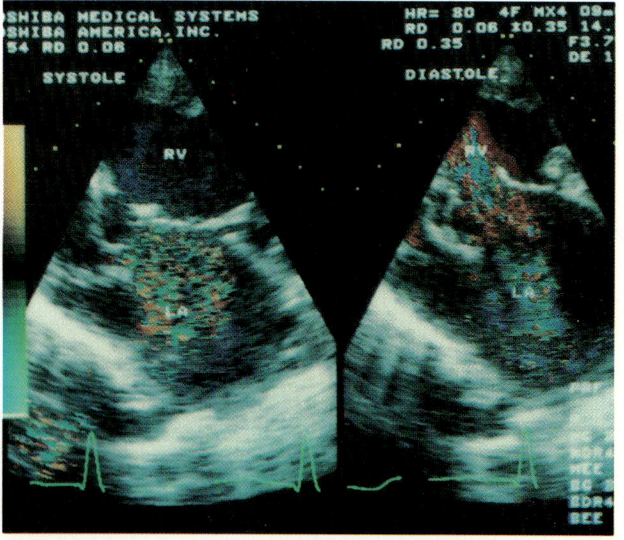

FIGURE 6-18—*Severe left atrioventricular valve regurgitation in a six-year-old boy with corrected transposition, intact ventricular septum, and Ebstein's malformation of the abnormal left-sided tricuspid valve. LA* = left atrium; RV = right ventricle.

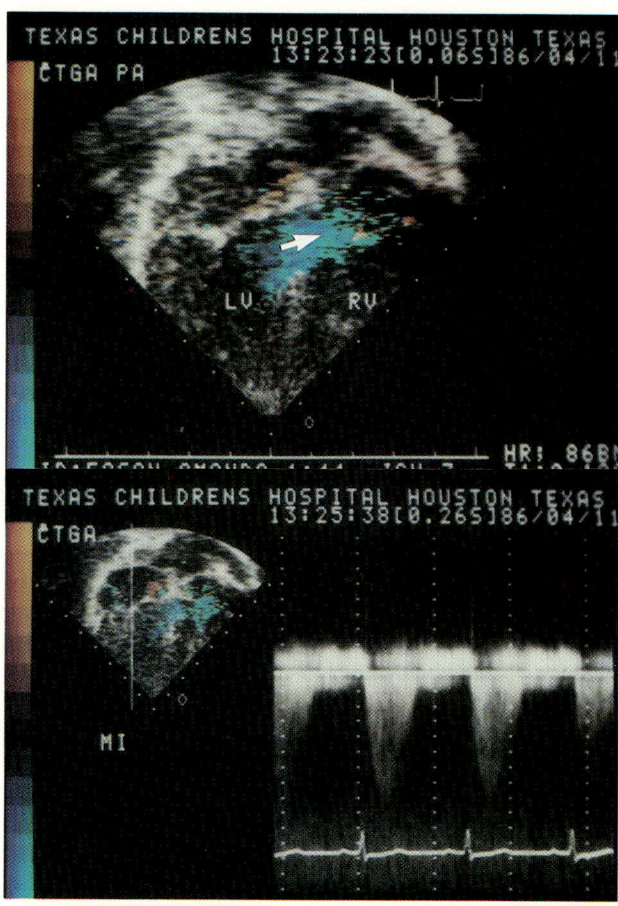

FIGURE 6-19—*Corrected transpostion in an infant with dextrocardia, pulmonary atresia, and a large ventricular septal defect (white arrow in upper panel). Doppler sampling of the right-sided mitral valve showed mild insufficiency and confirmed systemic pressure in the right-sided morphological left ventricle.*

References

1. Swensson RE, Sahn DJ, Valdes-Cruz LM: Color flow Doppler mapping in congenital heart disease. Echocardiography 2:545-549, 1985.
2. Omoto R: Color Atlas of Real-Time Two Dimensional Doppler Echocardiography. Tokyo, Sinden-To-Chiryosha, 1983.
3. Huhta JC, Seward JB, Tajik AJ, et al: Two-dimensional echocardiographic spectrum of univentricular atrioventricular connection. J Am Coll Cardiol 5:149-157, 1985.
4. Shiina A, Seward JB, Edwards WD, et al: Two-dimensional echocardiographic spectrum of Ebstein's anomaly: Detailed anatomic assessment. J Am Coll Cardiol 3:356-370, 1984.
5. Huhta JC, Danielson GK, Ritter DG, Ilstrup DM: Survival in atrioventricular discordance. Pediatr Cardiol 6:57-60, 1985.

Chapter 7

Intraoperative Examination

Don Hagler, M.D.

Intraoperative two-dimensional color Doppler represents a new and exciting area for development and refinement of this recently developed diagnostic modality.[1-2] In a preliminary study, we obtained intraoperative two-dimensional and color Doppler examinations in 30 patients with congenital heart disease (Table 7-I). The patients were examined intraoperatively immediately following cardiopulmonary bypass and surgical repair. In order to assess the sensitivity of the intraoperative findings we compared them to a complete two-dimensional Doppler color flow examination performed 10 to 14 days postoperatively. We used an Aloka 880 two-dimensional Doppler system with a standard, 5 MHz, phased- array transducer.

During the intraoperative examination, a long sterile plastic tube was used to encase the ultrasound transducer and cable. An ultrasound gel interface was used inside the sterile tube and sterile saline was placed over the exposed surface of the heart. With the standard 5 MHz transducer, imaging was limited to long-and short-axis views from the anterior surface of the heart without access to apical or inferior transducer positions. The late postoperative examinations were performed using the same instrument for color flow imaging but combined with a standard two-dimensional pulsed and continuous-wave Doppler examination using an ATL Ultramark 8 echocardiograph. Some continuous-wave Doppler examinations were obtained with an Irex III B nonimaging (Pedof) transducer.

TABLE 7-I

Intraoperative Two-dimensional Color Doppler

30 patients

12 female	mean age:	2.9 years
18 male	range:	2 weeks to 16 years

AV canal	3
TOF	5
PA	1
DOV	5
TGA	1
Dextrocardia, TGA	1
Truncus	2
Double inlet ventricle	2
VSD	7 (3 associated muscular VSD)
Aortic insufficiency	2
Ao-LV tunnel	1
Total	30

The intraoperative two-dimensional color flow examination allowed recognition of most of the residual hemodynamic abnormalities later demonstrated by the late postoperative echo study (Table 7- II). Small residual ventricular septal defects were observed in five patients during the intraoperative real-time study. One moderate-sized residual perimembranous ventricular septal defect was evident on late review of the intraoperative examination (Figure 7-1a). A later postoperative study confirmed the presence of a moderate-sized residual VSD with a high-velocity jet demonstrated with pulsed Doppler exam (Figure 7-1b). This patient subsequently required reoperation for the residual VSD. Residual small muscular ventricular septal defects were noted in two patients during the intraoperative examination (Figure 7-2).

Several factors contribute to failure to recognize small residual ventricular septal defects during the intraoperative examination. The most notable factor is the

TABLE 7-II

Color Imaging: Immediate Postop versus Late Findings

Correctly Observed
5 small VSD (2 muscular)
3 Aortic insufficiency (mild)
6 Tricuspid insufficiency (moderate)
5 Mitral insufficiency (mild)
1 Subaortic stenosis (mild)*
Missed
1 Perimembranous VSD (early)
2 Muscular VSDs (tiny)
1 Trivial AI (prosthetic)
1 Mild left AV valve insufficiency (DILV)
1 Tiny PDA
1 Tiny secundum ASD

*Early postop death

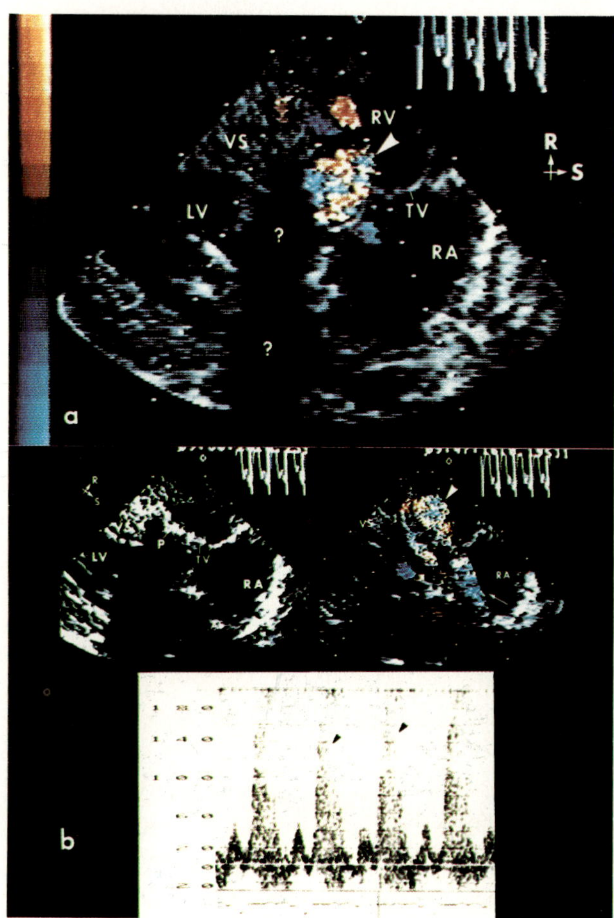

FIGURE 7-1—*(a) Intraoperative right ventricular inflow view of a one-year-old patient following ventricular septal defect repair. Note a large "echo dropout" posterior to the prosthetic patch indicated by question (?) marks. The arrowhead demonstrates turbulent high-velocity flow into the right ventricle (RV) consistent with a residual VSD. Also note the rapid heart rate of 150 beats/min shown by the ECG. (b) Composite showing intraoperative findings in the same patient and demonstrating a postoperative pulsed Doppler interrogation in the right ventricle of a high-velocity systolic jet consistent with a residual VSD. Note also a moderate tricuspid regurgitant jet coursing along the atrial septum. LV = left ventricle; RA = right atrium; R = right; S = superior; TV = tricuspid valve; VS = ventricular septum.*

extremely rapid heart rates encountered after cardiopulmonary bypass. Frequently, rates of 150 to 170 beats/min made timing of intracardiac flow events difficult (Figure 7-1a). Future developments, including faster frame rates with larger sector images, may improve recognition of flow events with such rapid heart rates. In addition, near-field imaging is compromised during the intraoperative examination. Because of the extremely narrow sector beam available for very near anterior structures, limited visibility of these structures was encountered. Also, the intensity of color flow signal and imaging was less in the near field. Thus, color flow imaging of very anterior structures such as the right ventricle is not ideal (Figure 7-3). Several attempts have made use of various offset devices (e.g., gel-filled bags) to allow improved imaging of anterior structures but as yet no commercially available intraoperative device is available.

With a very small near field available during the intraoperative examination, concomitant flow abnormalities with turbulence, as observed in Figure 7-3, may mask associated defects. Thus, in this example residual subpulmonary obstruction produces turbulent flow in the narrow right ventricular outflow tract. This turbulence masks the appearance of a tiny residual outlet ventricular septal defect which was more clearly detected and defined on later two-dimensional, pulsed, and continuous-wave Doppler study.

Following intracardiac repair of congenital defects, such as atrioventricular septal defects, the large echodense prosthetic patch may obscure more posterior structures (Figure 7-1a) such as the left ventricular outflow tract and left atrium. However, with more superior

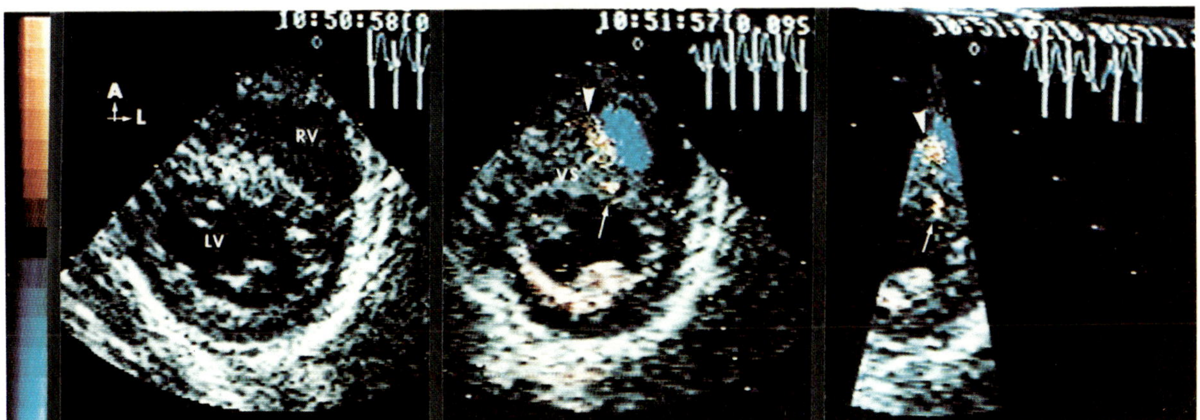

FIGURE 7-2—*Intraoperative parasternal short-axis view of a one-year-old patient following repair of tetralogy of Fallot. A tiny mid-septal muscular VSD is evident only with color flow imaging. The residual defect did not require further operative intervention. LV = left ventricle; RV = right ventricle.*

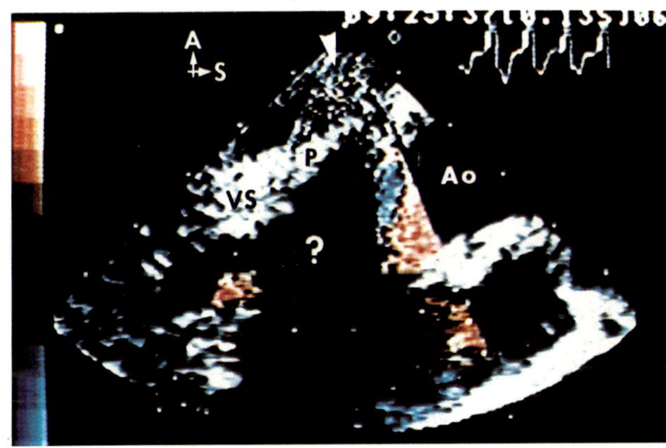

FIGURE 7-3—*Intraoperative long-axis scan in a two- year-old patient shows dense ventricular septal (VS) prosthetic patch (P). Note the turbulent (variance—green) flow in the RV anterior to the prosthetic patch. There was mild residual right ventricular outflow tract narrowing which seems to be responsible for the turbulent flow observed. However, a tiny outlet VSD was also detected on late postoperative examination. Note the echo dropout (?) posterior to the prosthetic patch. AO = aorta; A = anterior; S = superior.*

and lateral transducer placement, satisfactory color flow imaging of the mitral valve was obtained in all cases to assess residual mitral insufficiency (Figure 7-4).

In patients with valvular regurgitation, a pre-bypass intraoperative color flow assessment of the severity of regurgitation may be compared to the immediate postoperative findings. Figure 7-5a demonstrates the intraoperative pre-bypass findings in a three-year-old patient with a moderate-sized perimembranous VSD and severe mitral insufficiency. Figure 7-5b clearly demonstrates that the VSD patch has effectively closed the ventricular defect and repair of the mitral valve has reduced the mitral insufficiency to a mild degree of residual insufficiency.

The late postoperative examination using combined two-dimensional pulsed and continuous-wave Doppler study as well as color flow imaging allowed a precise assessment of the postoperative status and recognition of a number of residual postoperative findings that otherwise would have remained undetected. Combined use of multiple modalities allows the best assessment of such residual defects. Figure 7-6a demonstrates the presence of a typical small perimembranous residual ventricular septal defect in a patient following repair of tetralogy of Fallot. The 27-degree sector in the left panel allows a real-time demonstration of the left-to- right shunt at a frame rate of approximately 30 frames per second. Figure 7-6b demonstrates continuous-wave Doppler interrogation of the same residual ventricular septal defect. A maximum velocity of 3.2 meters per second was recorded, demonstrating a maximum instantaneous interventricular gradient of approximately 41 mmHg. Figure 7-6c demonstrates a moderate degree of tricuspid regurgitation observed in the same patient. Continuous-wave Doppler interrogation of the tricuspid regurgitation demonstrates a 3.0 meters per second systolic velocity predicting a 36 mmHg gradient and consistent with an expected right ventricular systolic pressure of approximately 50 mmHg.

In some cases, color flow imaging best demonstrated the residual defects although they were detectable in studies using pulsed or continuous-wave Doppler. For example, Figure 7-7 demonstrates residual patency of a tiny patent ductus arteriosus following surgical ligation. Pulsed Doppler interrogation of the main pulmonary artery demonstrates a very faint diastolic jet consistent with flow into the main pulmonary artery. However, more precise localization and interpretation of this jet was only possible with color Doppler. In summary, intraoperative color flow imaging was a sensitive and reliable method for intraoperative assessment of surgical repair of congential heart disease. These preliminary studies may help direct further development to improve some of the current limitations discussed above.

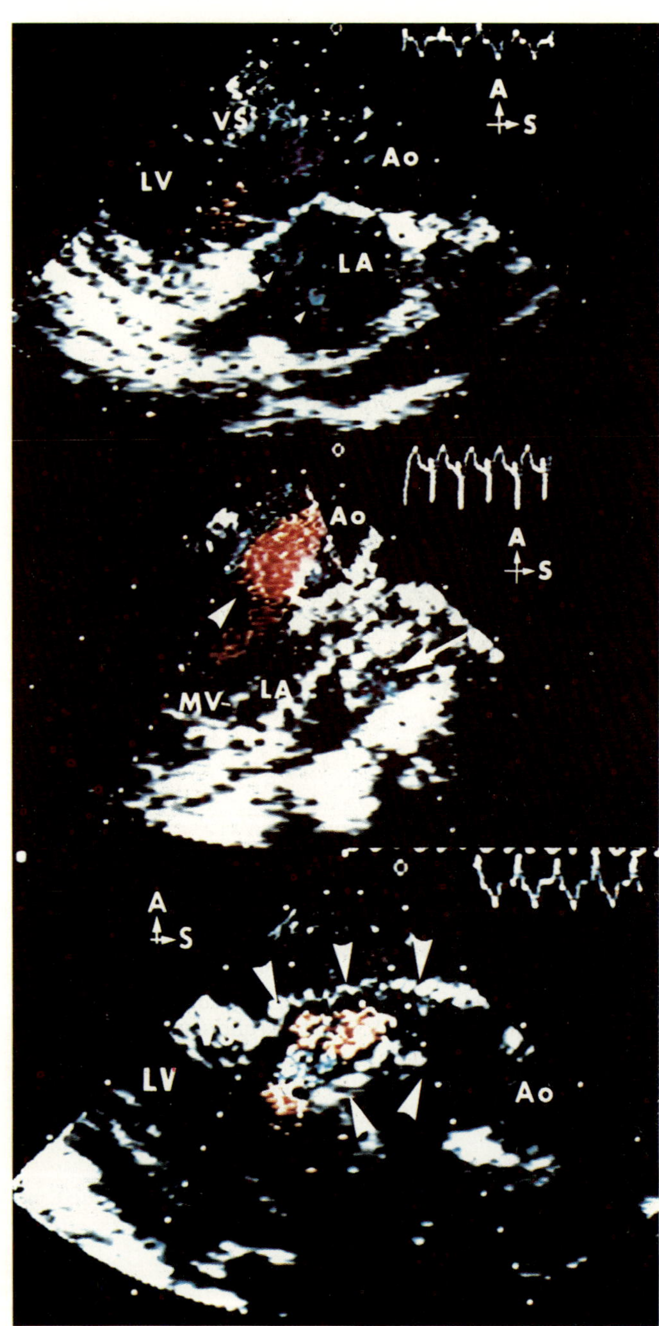

FIGURE 7-4—*(a) Intraoperative high long-axis scan of a six-year-old patient following repair of complete AV canal defect. A minimal degree of residual mitral valve insufficiency is observed. A = anterior; Ao = aorta; LA = left atrium; LV = left ventricle; S = superior; VS = ventricular septum. (b) Intraoperative high long-axis scan of a nine-month-old patient after repair of double outlet right ventricle demonstrates widely patent LV outflow to anterior aorta (Ao). In addition, the mitral valve (MV) is competent with no evidence of regurgitation into the left atrium (LA). The arrow points to systolic flow into the right pulmonary artery. A = anterior; S = superior. (c) Intraoperative high long-axis scan of a 15-month-old patient after repair of double outlet right ventricle with remote atrioventricular septal defect. Note the long course of intraventricular tunnel (arrowheads) from the left ventricle (LV) to the aorta (Ao). Only mild aliasing is observed within the conduit, suggesting minimally increased velocity and no significant obstruction to aortic flow. A = anterior; S = superior; VS = ventricular septum.*

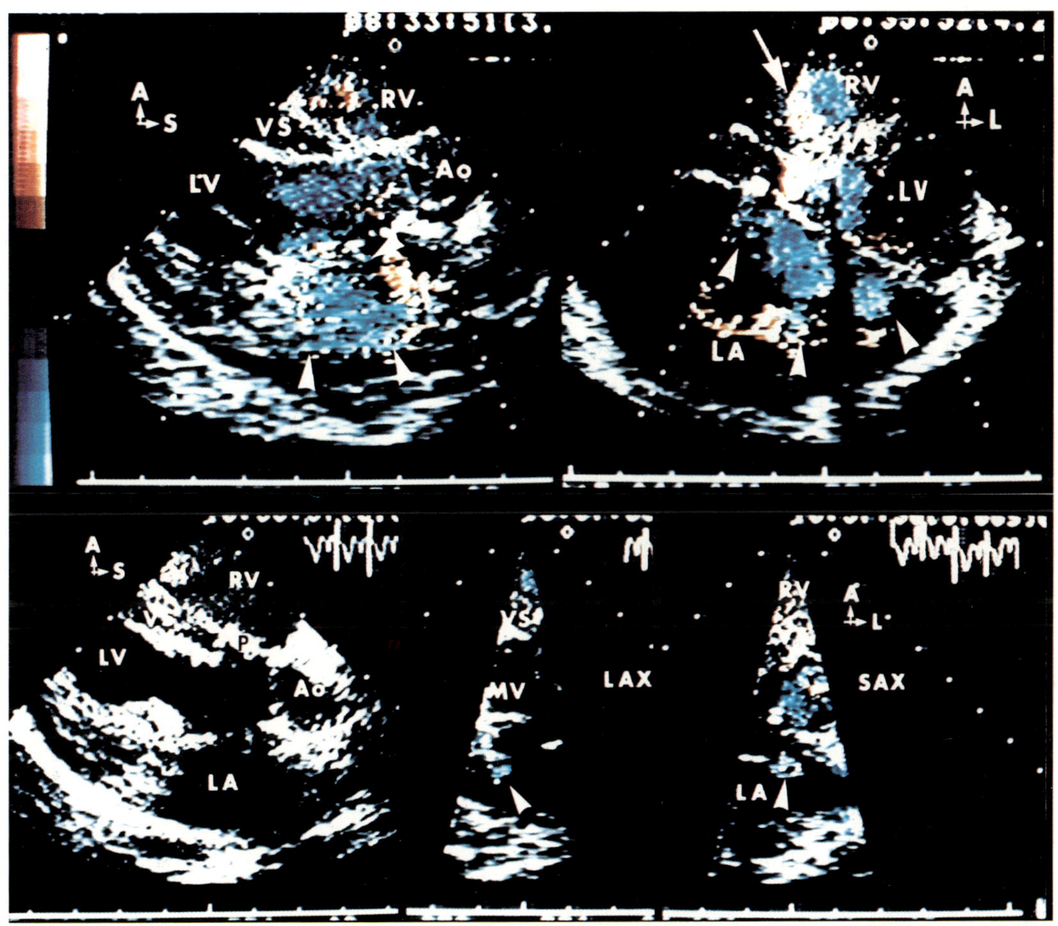

FIGURE 7-5—Intraoperative long (left) and short (right) axis scans in a three-year-old patient prior to cardiopulmonary bypass demonstrate preoperative findings of small perimembranous VSD (arrow) and severe mitral valve insufficiency (arrowheads). (b) Intraoperative long (left and middle) and short (right) axis scans of the same patient immediately following surgical correction demonstrate a mild degree of residual mitral insufficiency with a tiny regurgitant jet into the left atrium (left). No residual VSD is evident. A = anterior; L = left; S = superior; Ao = aorta; La = left atrium; LV = left ventricle; RV = right ventricle; VS = ventricular septum; LA = long axis; SA = short axis; P = patch.

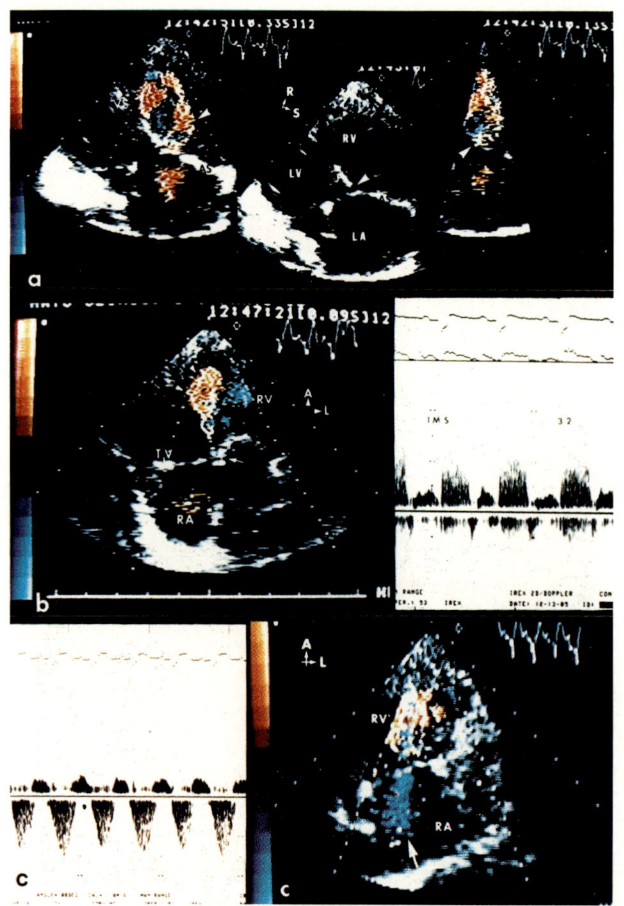

FIGURE 7-6—*(a) Postoperative color flow examination of a two-year-old patient following repair of tetralogy of Fallot. A small perimembranous VSD is evident (arrowhead) The left panel demonstrates the left-to-right shunt in real time at 30 frames per second. (b) Postoperative short-axis scan in the same patient demonstrates the location of the VSD near the tricuspid valve (TV) with continuous-wave Doppler. The left panel demonstrates the continuous-wave Doppler velocity recorded with a maximum velocity of 3.2 meters per second. This would be consistent with a maximum instantaneous LV/RV pressure gradient of 41 mmHg. (c) Another short-axis scan in the same patient demonstrates a moderate regurgitant jet of tricuspid insufficiency. Continuous-wave Doppler study reveals a velocity of 3.0 meters per second consistent with an estimated right ventricular systolic pressure of approximately 50 mmHg.*

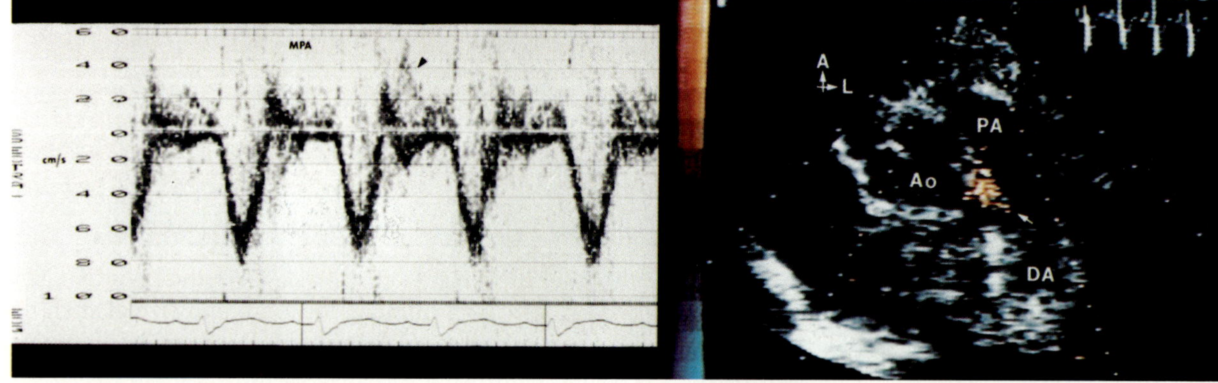

FIGURE 7-7—*Pulsed Doppler examination in a two-year-old patient following repair of VSD and PDA ligation. Diastolic positive flow (arrowhead) is detected in the main pulmonary artery. Color flow imaging clearly demonstrated the origin of the diastolic flow from the area of the ligated ductus. Ao = aorta; DA = descending aorta; PA = pulmonary artery; A = anterior; L = left.*

References

1. Goldman ME: Intraoperative 2-dimensional echocardiography: New application of an old technique. J Am Coll Cardiol 7:374-382, 1986.
2. Takamoto S, Kyo S, et al: Sponsored by MJ Buckley. Intraoperative color flow mapping by real-time two-dimensional Doppler echocardiography for evaluation of valvular and congenital heart disease and vascular disease. J Thorac Cardiovasc Surg 90:802-812, 1985.

Chapter 8

Postoperative Congenital Heart Disease

Daniel J. Murphy, Jr., M.D., and Victoria E. Judd, M.D.

Surgery for correction or palliation of congenital heart defects invariably changes the flow patterns in the heart and great vessels. In many instances, surgery eliminates abnormalities of flow; however, with equal frequency new flow disturbances are created or an alteration of the original abnormality occurs. For example, the surgical relief of valvular stenosis results in a decrease in the transvalvular velocities. However, a mild flow disturbance persists and frequently valvular insufficiency is created. Therefore, the goal of color flow mapping in the postoperative patient following surgery for congenital heart disease is to confirm that the desired alterations in flow patterns have occurred and to detect the presence of any new flow disturbances. As with a preoperative patient, a careful systematic evaluation of systolic and diastolic flow at each location in the heart and great vessels is necessary for an accurate assessment of the patient's hemodynamic status.

Tetralogy of Fallot

Corrective surgery for tetralogy of Fallot involves patch closure of the ventricular septal defect, closure of any atrial septal defect, and relief of right ventricular outflow tract obstruction. Color Doppler is helpful in the detection of residual ventricular septal defects or patch leaks (Figure 8-1). Such lesions are best demonstrated in the short-axis or modified four-chamber views as jets transversing the ventricular septum from left to right. These systolic jets are generally high-velocity and color Doppler can be used to direct continuous-wave examination for the determination of peak instantaneous velocity.

Although successful surgery for tetralogy of Fallot relieves right ventricular outflow tract obstruction, a flow disturbance remains that may be detectable with color flow mapping (Figure 8-2). In addition, unless a prosthetic valve is inserted, there is usually pulmonary regurgitation. This diastolic flow toward the transducer in the right ventricular outflow tract is easily demonstrated by color flow mapping (Figures 8-2 and 8-3). Tricuspid regurgitation is also detectable in the majority of patients following surgical repair of tetralogy of Fallot. This is particularly true when right ventricular pressure remains elevated because of residual right ventricular outflow tract obstruction. Peripheral pulmonary stenosis is a significant postoperative abnormality in some patients with tetralogy of Fallot. Unfortunately, because of the angle between the axis of flow and the ultrasound beam, acceleration due to pulmonary branch stenosis is generally not detectable using color Doppler methods. In patients in whom an extracardiac conduit has been placed for relief of pulmonary atresia, obstruction within the conduit or at its proximal or distal ends will result in detectable acceleration of flow and turbulence.

Ventricular Septal Defect

In the early postoperative period, small leaks around the ventricular septal defect patch are not uncommon. These are discrete high-velocity systolic jets that are easily detectable with color flow mapping. By 72 hours following surgery, the detection of systolic flow across the ventricular septum indicates a residual ventricular septal defect. The number, location, and size of such defects can be assessed using color Doppler.[1,2] This is particularly important in the patient with multiple ventricular septal defects or with muscular defects in the trabecular portion of the muscular septum. Scanning should be performed in several planes, including the parasternal short-axis and the modified four-chamber view, and subcostal views (Figure 8-4).

Tricuspid regurgitation is not unusual following surgical repair of ventricular septal defects, particularly when this is accomplished through the tricuspid valve. Significant tricuspid regurgitation is rare. The detection of tricuspid regurgitation with color Doppler is useful as a guide for the use of continuous- wave Doppler for the detection of peak systolic velocity in the regurgitant

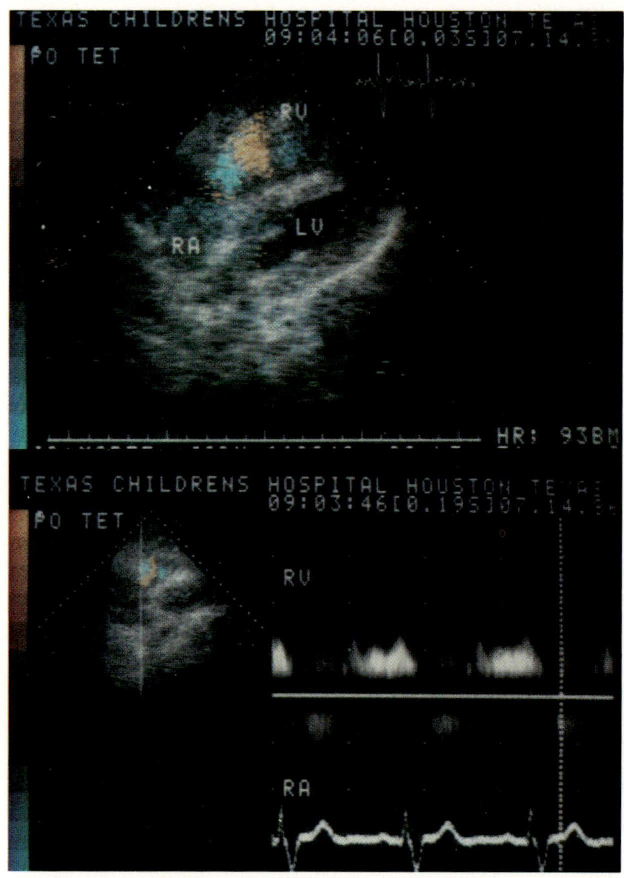

FIGURE 8-1—*Postoperative patient with tetralogy of Fallot with systolic murmurs. In the upper panel a short-axis scan gated in systole demonstrates a jet (orange color) into the right ventricle through a residual ventricular septal defect. In the lower panel continuous-wave Doppler confirmation of a tricuspid regurgitation jet is shown (right). In this case precise detection and characterization of the systolic flow disturbances requires real-time imaging, careful pulsed Doppler interrogation, color flow mapping, and continuous-wave Doppler examination. Complete examination clarifies the clinical findings.*

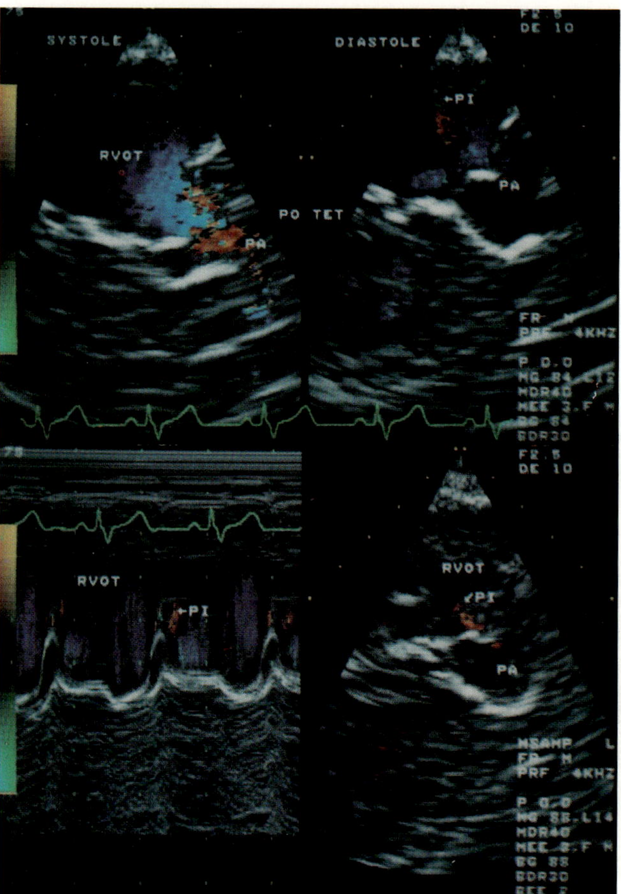

FIGURE 8-2—*Postoperative tetralogy of Fallot with residual pulmonary stenosis and pulmonary insufficiency. The upper panel demonstrates flow in the pulmonary outflow tract in systole (left) and diastole (right). Systolic flow is disturbed resulting in an orange-speckled color in the outflow tract and main pulmonary artery. In diastole there is flow of blood toward the transducer seen as a red jet. The lower panel illustrates the M-mode appearance of the pulmonary insufficiency jet. The jet was first detected using real-time color Doppler (right) and then an M-mode cursor was placed through the jet.*

jet. This is helpful in determining right ventricular pressure estimation.

Atrioventricular Canal Defect

Surgery for atrioventricular canal defect is aimed at closing the interatrial and interventricular communications and reconstruction of the atrioventricular valves. In the ideal situation there would be no atrial or ventricular septal defects postoperatively. In addition, the right and left atrioventricular valves would be neither stenotic nor insufficient. In fact, however, residual flow disturbances are common following surgery for complete AV canal defect. The most frequently encountered abnormalities are those of mild atrioventricular valve regurgitation. This is easily documented with color Doppler (Figures 8-5 and 8-6).[3] As with other complex lesions involving closure of a ventricular septal defect, postoperative color flow mapping can detect residual VSDs in patients with atrioventricular canal lesions (Figure 8-6).

The complete examination includes assessment of flow across all four intracardiac valves. This is extremely important following repair of AV canal. Obstruction to left ventricular outflow may occur postoperatively. For this reason, flow should be examined in the subaortic and aortic areas. In addition, distortion of the aortic valve occasionally will occur secondary to placement of the ventricular septal component of the patch. This in turn

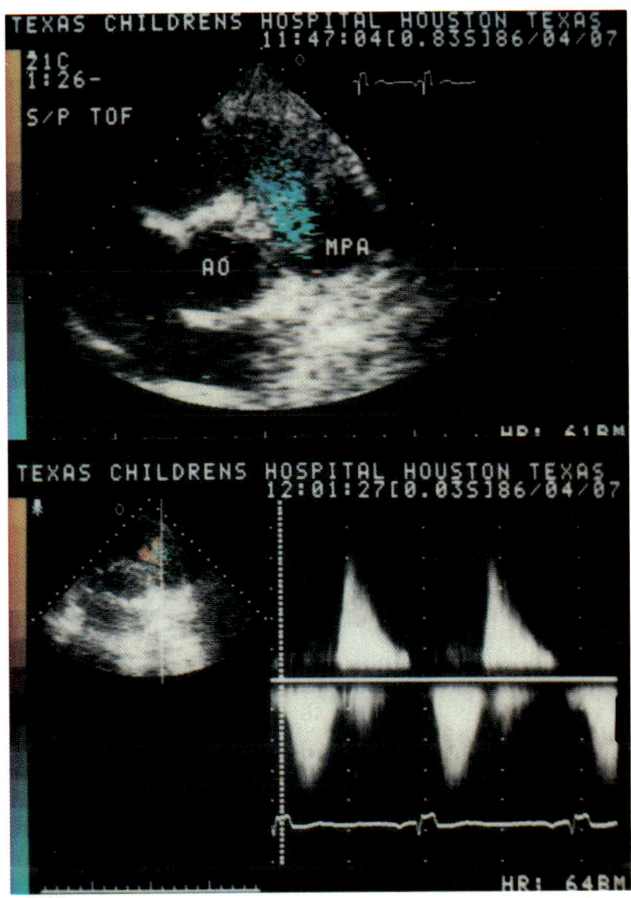

FIGURE 8-3—*Postoperative tetralogy of Fallot with pulmonary insufficiency without stenosis. Upper panel: pulmonary flow is demonstated by systolic gating. The color is relatively uniform without evidence of acceleration or flow disturbance. Lower panel: a diastolic jet toward the transducer has been detected during real-time scanning (left). A continuous-wave cursor is phased through the outflow tract and main pulmonary artery. The continuous-wave tracing (right) demonstrates relatively low-velocity systolic flow (peak velocity = 1.8 meters per second) and a pulmonary insufficiency jet in diastole.*

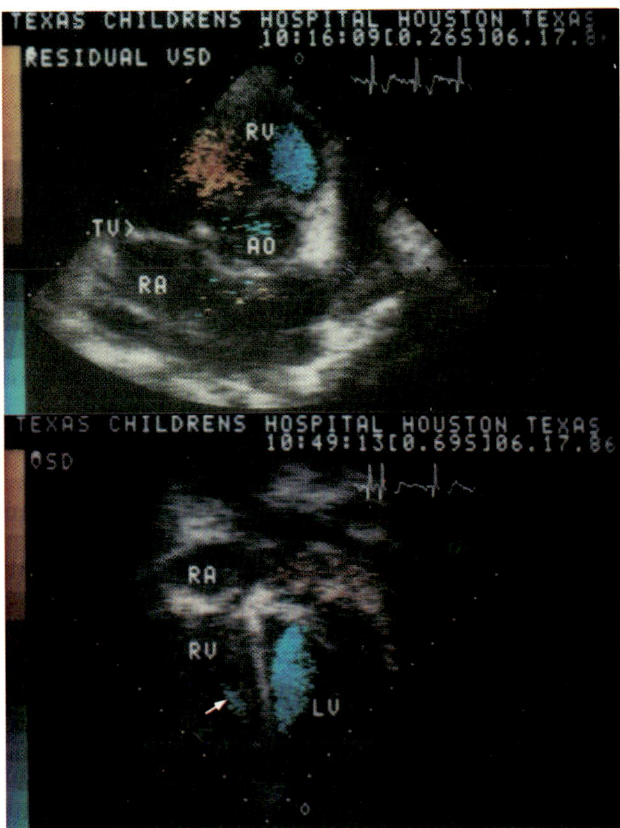

FIGURE 8-4—*Postoperative ventricular septal defect with residual shunt. In the upper panel a parasternal short-axis scan demonstrates a systolic jet (orange) toward the transducer into the right ventricle. The jet is more prominent than those from a patch leak and represents a residual septal defect. In the lower panel an apical four-chamber scan demonstrates normal left ventricular outflow and a systolic jet (blue) in the right ventricle from a residual apical muscular ventricular septal defect.*

may produce aortic insufficiency. Therefore, postoperative diastolic gating of aortic flow should be performed.

Transposition of the Great Arteries

The most significant hemodynamic abnormality encountered in patients following a Mustard or Senning repair for transposition of the great arteries is obstruction to venous flow. This may occur on the pulmonary or systemic side and at the entrance of the veins to the atrium or at the midportion of the baffle (Figures 8-7 and 8-8). Therefore, careful flow mapping is required in the pulmonary and systemic veins, as well as in the atrium through the midportions of the baffle. A two-dimensional echocardiographic appearance of narrowing with Doppler evidence of increased velocity should guide the examiner to use continuous- wave Doppler to determine peak velocities. Venous inflow velocities above 1.5 meters per second strongly suggest obstructed venous flow.

Left ventricular outflow tract obstruction is not uncommon in patients with transposition of the great arteries and discrete stenosis can develop in the postoperative period. Therefore evaluation of flow in the left ventricular outflow tract is important in the postoperative examination of the patient with transposition of the great arteries.

Following arterial switch procedures, the major area of concern is the presence of aortic stenosis or insufficiency. This is particularly true in the patient with previous pulmonary artery banding in whom the left-sided semilunar valve annulus is dilated.

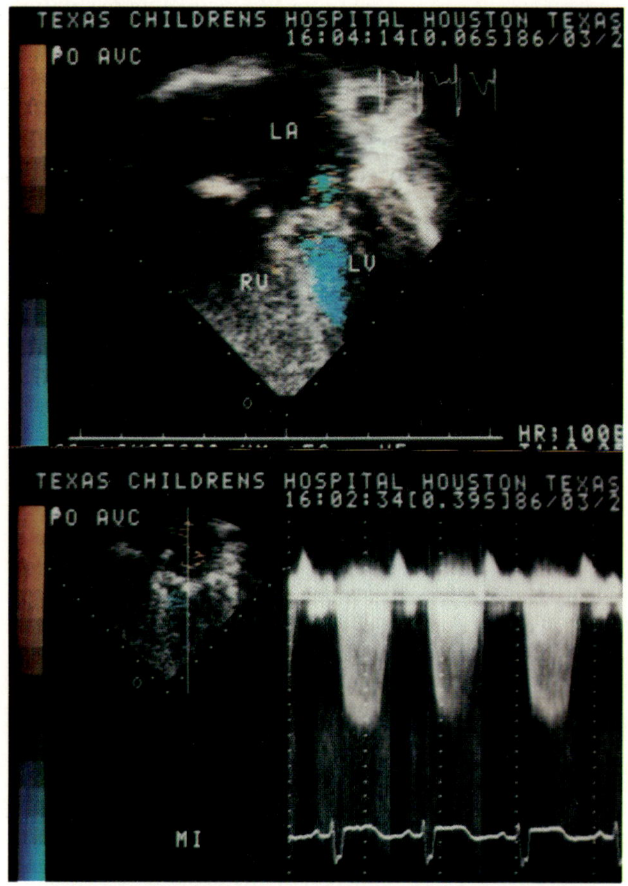

FIGURE 8-5—*Postoperative atrioventricular canal defect with mitral regurgitation. In the upper panel a modified apical four-chamber view demonstrates a systolic jet into the left atrium from the left ventricle. Normal left ventricular systolic outflow is present along the ventricular septum. In the lower panel a continuous-wave cursor has been placed through the mitral valve (left) and the continuous-wave Doppler tracing (right) demonstrates high-velocity (4.3 meters per second) systolic flow away from the transducer due to mitral regurgitation. Unlike the posterior and lateral jets of rheumatic mitral regurgitation, the jet associated with endocardial cushion defect frequently is directed medially toward the atrial septum.*

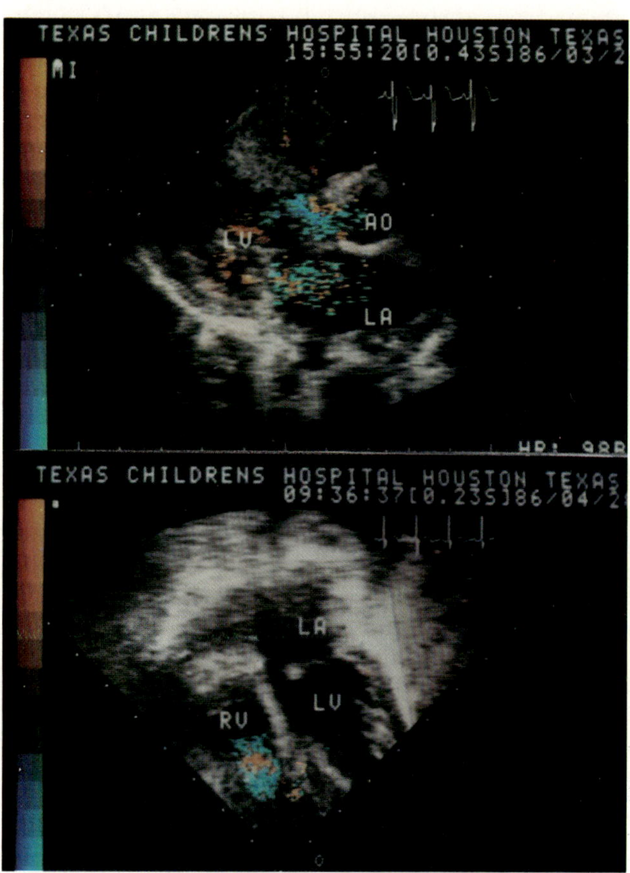

FIGURE 8-6—*Postoperative atrioventricular canal defect with mitral regurgitation and residual ventricular septal defect. In the upper panel a systolic jet of mitral regurgitation is detected in the left atrium in the parasternal long-axis view. In the lower panel a modified apical four-chamber view in systole demonstrates a residual ventricular septal defect (an orange jet through the septum into the right ventricle). Visualization of the jet can be used to direct continuous-wave Doppler estimation of right ventricular pressure.*

Truncus Arteriosus

The repair of truncus arteriosus achieves many of the same goals as that of tetralogy of Fallot. The ventricular septal defect must be patched and continuity between the right ventricle and pulmonary arteries established. In addition, there is the added difficulty of truncal valve stenosis or insufficiency. Therefore, careful flow mapping should be performed of the ventricular septal defect area, as well as of the truncal valve. Careful gating to systole for VSD or truncal stenosis detection and to diastole for truncal insufficiency will assist in the diagnosis of residual flow disturbances.

As with other lesions involving closure of ventricular septal defect or right ventricular outflow tract obstruction, in truncus arteriosus the presence of tricuspid regurgitation is particularly important both in the functional assessment of the right ventricle and in the estimation of right ventricular pressure. Careful examination of the tricuspid valve and right atrium should therefore be performed using color flow mapping in an attempt to detect tricuspid insufficiency.

Aortopulmonary Shunts

A variety of aortopulmonary communications have been used to increase pulmonary blood flow as a pallia-

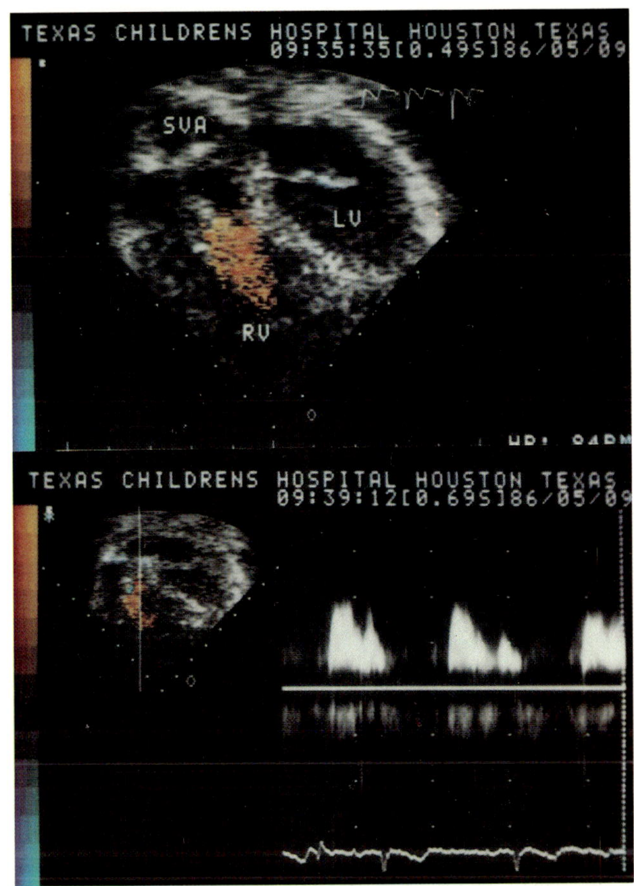

FIGURE 8-7—*Transposition of the great arteries following a Senning procedure. Imaging in the modified apical four-chamber view (upper panel) and continuous-wave Doppler (lower panel) demonstrate normal right ventricular inflow velocities. Peak velocity is 1 meter per second in diastole and there is no systolic flow, thus excluding tricuspid regurgitation.*

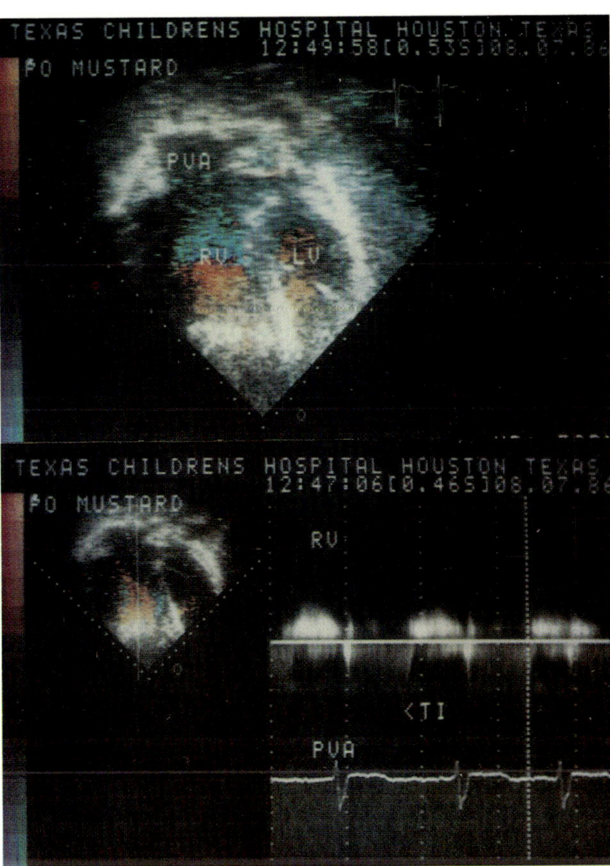

FIGURE 8-8—*Transposition of the great arteries following a Mustard procedure. Diastolic inflow into both ventricles from the apical four-chamber view (upper panel) reveals no evidence of high-velocity diastolic flow. Continuous-wave Doppler (lower panel) confirms low-velocity right ventricular inflow in diastole and demonstrates tricuspid regurgitation in systole.*

tive approach to cyanotic congenital heart disease. With careful attention to imaging planes and technique, flow in shunts can be documented with color flow mapping (Figures 8-9 and 8-10). With low pulmonary artery pressure, flow is generally of relatively high velocity in the shunt and therefore easily detected with color flow techniques. However, elevated pulmonary pressure may result in low shunt flow velocity, making the differentiation between shunt occlusion and elevated pulmonary pressure difficult. In such an instance pulsed Doppler should be used to resolve the dilemma.

Tricuspid Atresia, Single Ventricle (Fontan Procedure)

The Fontan procedure and its modifications attempt to eliminate communications between the pulmonary and systemic circulations. Typically the right atrium is connected to the pulmonary arteries with or without the use of a conduit. However, occasionally a rudimentary right ventricle will be incorporated into the right side of the circulation. In most cases, flow on the right side of the heart is of low velocity and has a "venous" pattern. Significant acceleration of flow at any point suggests the presence of obstruction. Therefore, careful flow mapping from the vena cava to the main pulmonary artery is helpful. Flow on the right side of the heart should be examined in both systole and diastole. Incorporation of the right ventricle or obstruction to pulmonary flow may result in retrograde flow, particularly in systole. This would be an indication of an unsatisfactory hemodynamic situation (Figures 8-11 and 8-12).

Any residual communication between the pulmonary and systemic circuits may produce volume overload and hemodynamically compromise the patient follow-

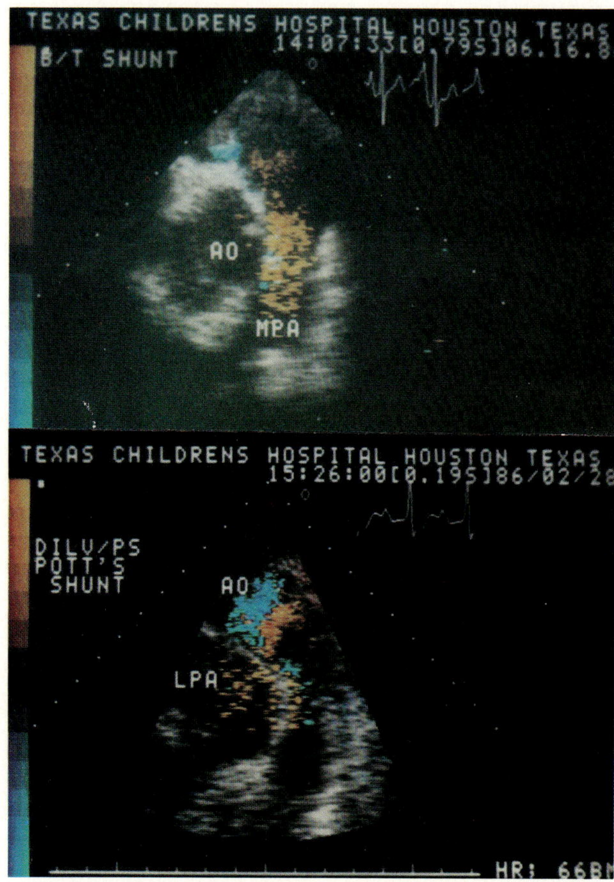

FIGURE 8-9—*Upper panel: Blalock-Taussig shunt. Parasternal short-axis scan gated in diastole demonstrates turbulent flow filling the main pulmonary artery. The flow in the shunt is not demonstrated in this view and is best seen from the suprasternal notch. Lower panel: Pott's shunt from the left pulmonary artery to the descending aorta.*

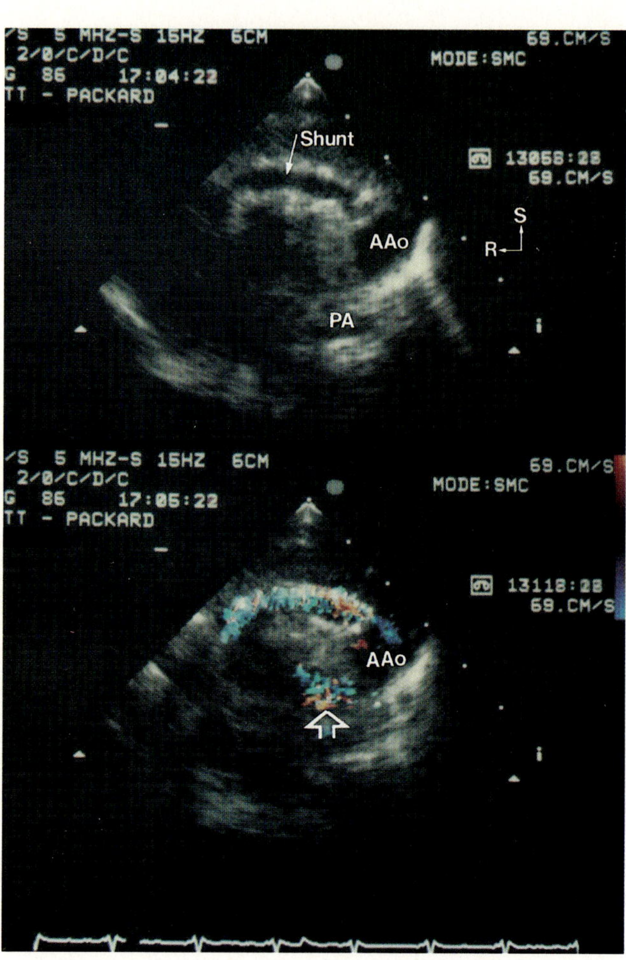

FIGURE 8-10—*Goretex® aortopulmonary shunt. Imaging (upper panel) and color Doppler (lower panel) from the suprasternal notch demonstrate a 5 mm Goretex® shunt from ascending aorta to right pulmonary artery. Flow is phasic and turbulent in the shunt and in the pulmonary artery.*

ing the Fontan operation. Therefore, the detection of significant ventricular septal defects or atrial septal defects is important. In general, right atrial pressure is elevated and therefore atrial leaks occur from right to left. These may be difficult to detect with color flow mapping because of their location. Ventricular septal defects on the other hand are generally of high velocity and should be easy to detect (Figure 8-13). In patients with two atrioventricular valves, the Fontan operation frequently involves patch closure of the right- sided AV valve (Figure 8-14). Incomplete closure of this valve will result in a left-to-right shunt. This high-velocity jet is usually directed into the right atrium and should be detected with careful flow mapping of the right atrium with systolic gating.

Glenn anastomosis (superior vena cava to right pulmonary artery shunt) is used to increase pulmonary blood flow as a palliative approach for tricuspid atresis (Figure 8-15).

Severe mitral regurgitation is usually considered a contraindication to the Fontan procedure. Occasionally, however, patients with mild mitral regurgitation undergo this operation. Any significant mitral regurgitation in the postoperative period will result in severe hemodynamic compromise. Therefore, careful color flow mapping of the mitral valve is useful.

Pulmonary Artery Banding

Pulmonary artery banding is performed in selected patients as a palliative maneuver for reducing pulmonary artery flow. Two-dimensional echocardiography can be used to image the band area in the parasternal short-axis, suprasternal, and subcostal views. Distal obstruction of the right or left pulmonary artery can be detected. The efficacy of the pulmonary artery band is accurately

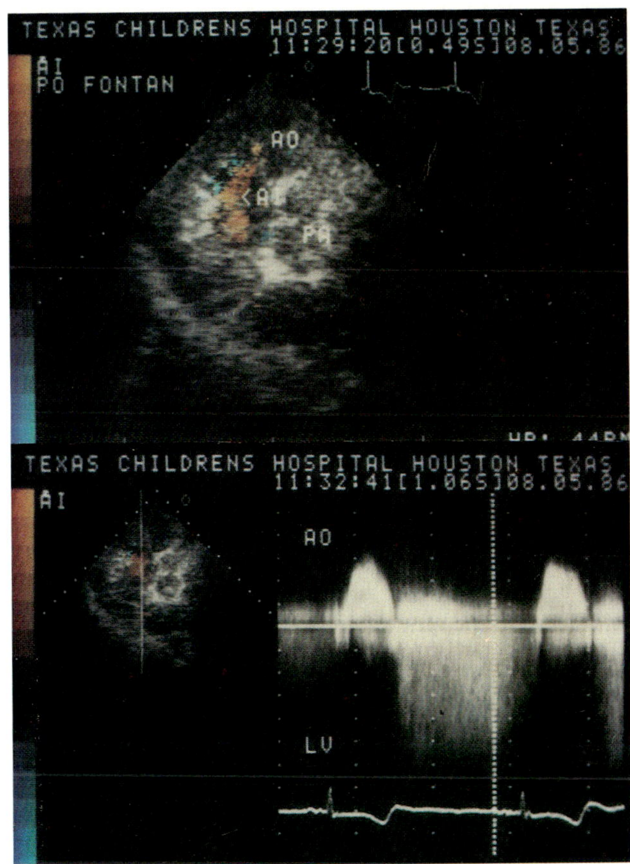

FIGURE 8-11—*Single ventricle, transposition of the great arteries, postoperative Fontan procedure with aortic regurgitation. Diastolic imaging (upper panel) and continuous-wave Doppler (lower panel) demonstrate the presence of aortic regurgitation.*

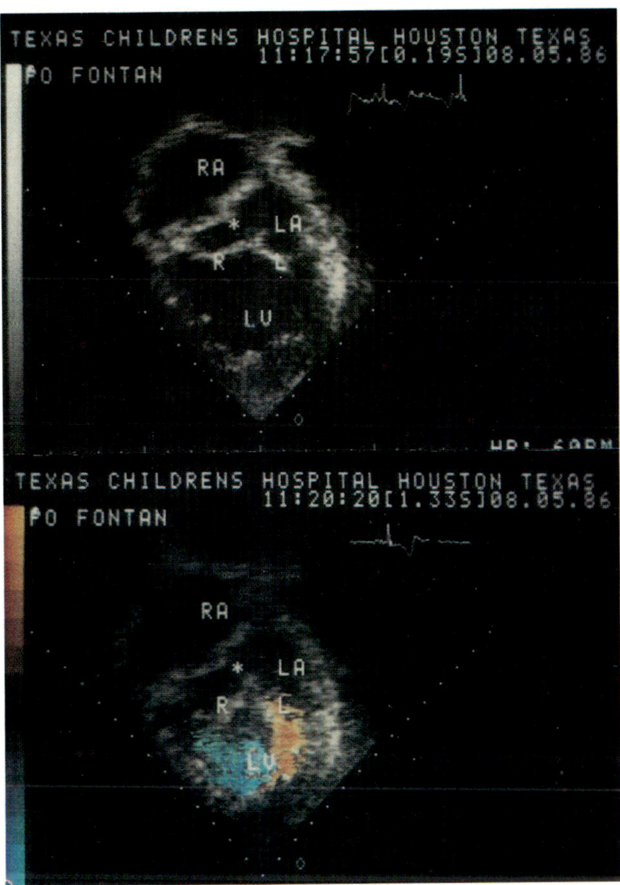

FIGURE 8-12—*Double inlet left ventricle, postoperative Fontan procedure. Repair included an atrial battle that directed pulmonary venous flow into both atrioventricular valves and anastamosis between right atrium and main pulmonary artery. In the lower panel diastolic ventricular inflow is demonstrated. No flow is detected in the right atrium or left atrium because of the low flow velocities and distance from the transducer.* * = *coronary sinus.*

estimated by pulsed and continuous-wave Doppler. Color Doppler is useful for imaging of the jet direction for continuous and pulsed Doppler evaluation and detection of distal obstruction in the right or left pulmonary artery (Figures 8-16 and 8-17). In this case the mosaic pattern seen across the pulmonary artery band will change to another color as a result of velocity changes if a high-pressure gradient across the pulmonary artery band is present and aliasing just proximal to the band appears.

Prosthetic Valves

Two-dimensional real-time Doppler color flow mapping techniques have shown obvious application in the evaluation of native valve structure and function. These techniques are in their infancy in the evaluation of the function of both normal and abnormal valvular prostheses. Color Doppler has certain capabilities that provide a way of assessing the function of prosthetic valves. In addition to providing information about turbulence, direction, and velocity of blood flow, it also provides a spatial orientation to blood flow patterns.

Prosthetic valves may be classified according to their number of leaflets or occluders, according to the types of materials used for their manufacture or according to their flow characteristics. Typed according to their flow characteristic, there are three types: (1) valves with peripheral flow (ball and cage, disc and cage): the Starr-Edwards is the most common type; (2) the eccentric flow valve (tilting disc), of which the Bjork Shiley and St. Jude are the most common; and (3) valves with central flow (homografts, autographs, bioprosthetic valves).

The diagnosis of prosthetic valve dysfunction is often difficult and requires the integration of many avail-

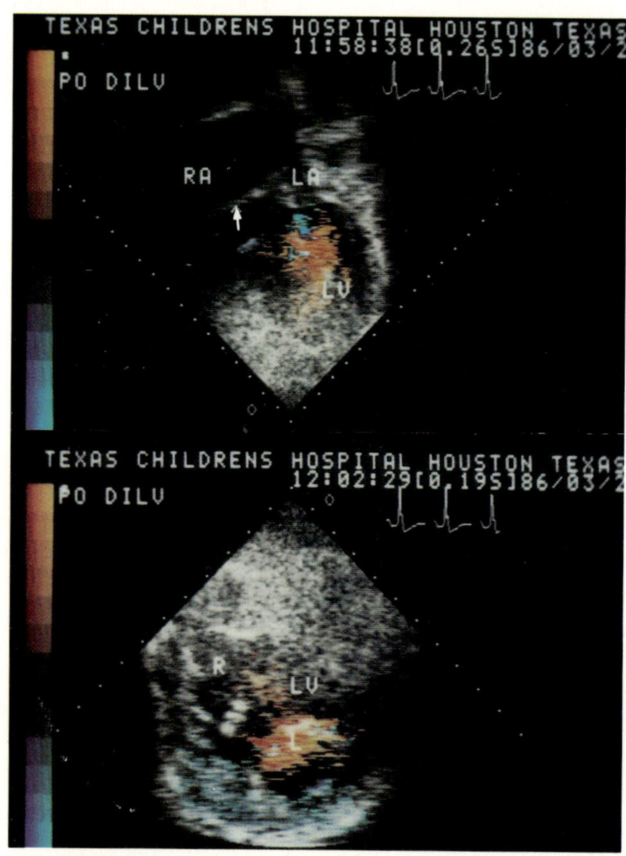

FIGURE 8-13—*Tricuspid atresia, transposition of the great arteries, postoperative Fontan procedure. Two parasternal views demonstrate flow through a ventricular septal defect in systole. The defect appears small and the color flow mapping can be used to guide continuous-wave Doppler estimation of pressure gradient across the defect.*

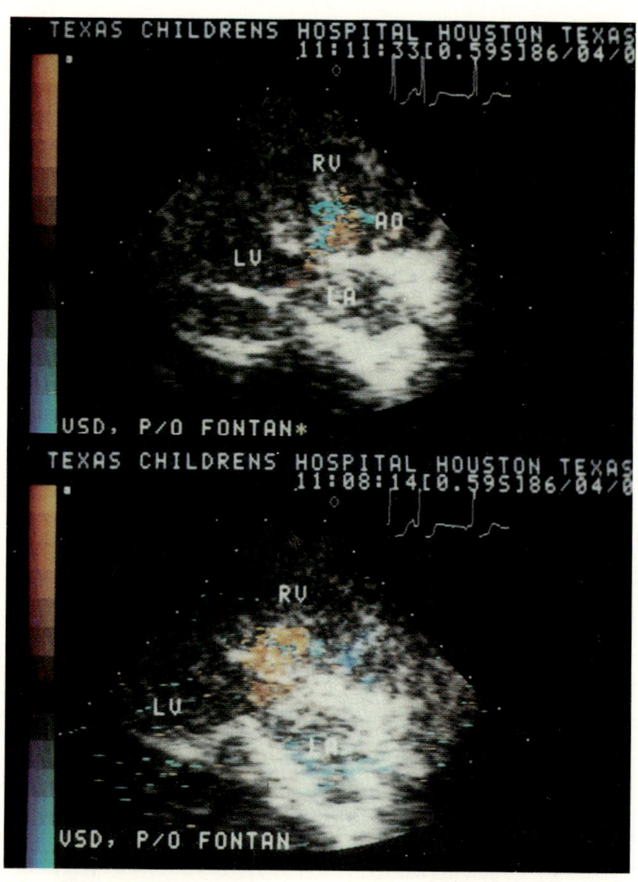

FIGURE 8-14—*Double inlet left ventricle, postoperative Fontan procedure. Repair included patch closure of the tricuspid valve. Diastolic flow mapping in the apical (upper panel) and parasternal short-axis (lower panel) views demonstrates unobstructed flow through the left atrioventricular valve and no apparent flow through the right. Patch leak can result in a significant bidirectional shunt and hemodynamic compromise.*

able methods. M-mode, two-dimensional, continuous-wave, and pulsed Doppler echocardiography have limitations in the evaluation of prosthetic valve dysfunction. One of the major difficulties is that Doppler frequency shifts can be detected only along the one-dimensional line of the cursor. This limits the examiner's ability to define the true three-dimensional spatial orientation of the jet.

Each type of valve has its own velocity flow profile. Aliasing may occur with normally functioning prosthetic heart valves (Figure 8-18), especially the peripheral flow and eccentric flow valves. Peripheral flow valves produce a ten centimeter cone- shaped velocity profile with both a central and a peripheral vortex. Eccentric flow valves produce elliptical flow profiles from both the major and minor orifices (Figure 8-18). Central flow valves produce a central pyramidal flow profile with circumferential vortices.[4]

Prosthetic valve malfunction observed with Doppler color flow studies includes regurgitant flow, perivalvular and intrinsic valve regurgitation, stenosis of the prosthetic valve, and abnormal leaflet, ball, or disc motion.

Color Doppler offers significant advantages in the noninvasive evaluation of valvular regurgitation because of its two- dimensional flow mapping capacity. This improves the sensitivity for detection of mild regurgitation, eccentric regurgitant jets, and multivalvular regurgitation. Color Doppler allows for grading of the regurgitant jet by providing a two-dimensional image of the jet's width and area.[5,6] Color Doppler can be used in the immediate postoperative period to assess prosthetic valve function detecting multivalvular dysfunction and perivalvular and intrinsic valve regurgitation (Figures 8-19, 8-20, and 8-21).

Doppler can be used to detect disturbed high-velocity flow jets across prosthetic valves and can allow for spatial orientation information to guide continuous-wave Doppler estimation of transvalvular gradients.[7]

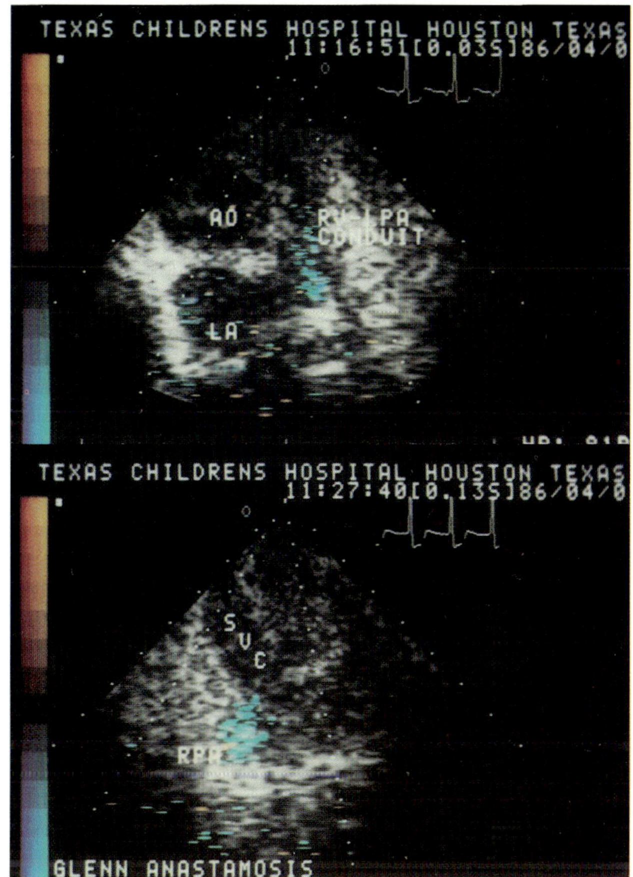

FIGURE 8-15—*Tricuspid atresia, postoperative right ventricle to left pulmonary artery conduit, and Glenn anastamosis. Systolic flow is demonstrated in the conduit in the parasternal view (upper panel). Flow is also demonstrated in the right pulmonary artery near the anastamosis with the superior vena cava from the suprasternal notch (lower panel).*

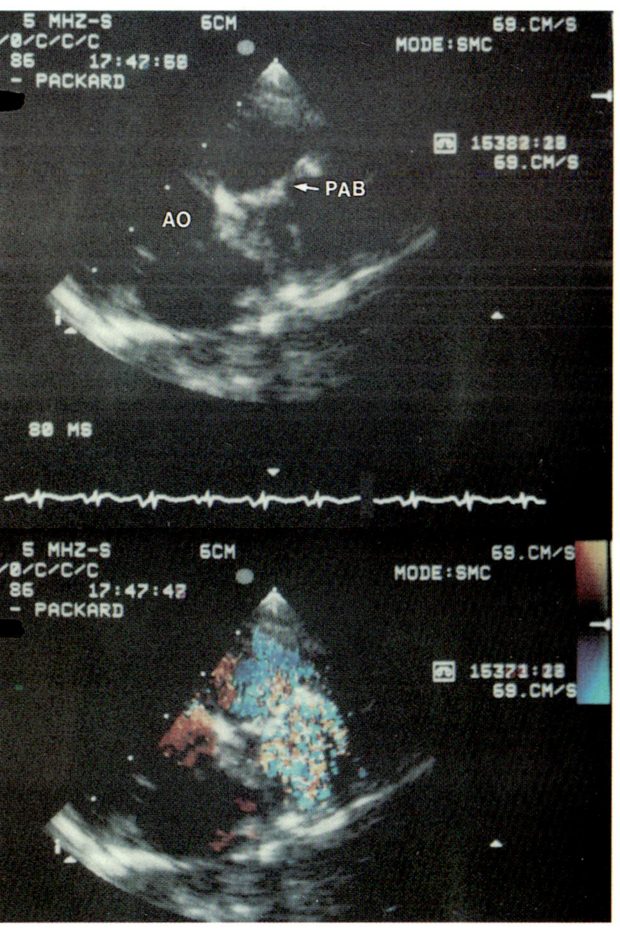

FIGURE 8-16—*Pulmonary artery band. Two- dimensional imaging demonstrates the location of the band on the main pulmonary artery (upper panel). Color flow mapping demonstrates acceleration of flow proximal to the band and disturbed flow distal to the band (lower panel).*

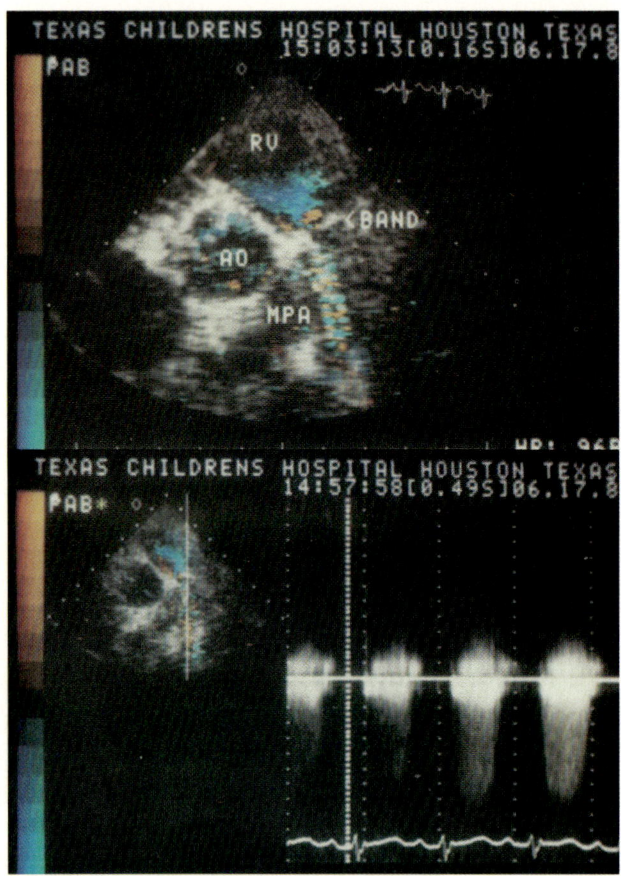

FIGURE 8-17—*Pulmonary artery band. Color flow mapping (upper panel) demonstrates a systolic jet in the center of the main pulmonary artery and is used to guide continuous-wave Doppler (lower panel). The high-velocity systolic jet (4.6 meters per second) can be used to calculate the pulmonary artery pressure and confirm the adequacy of pulmonary artery banding.*

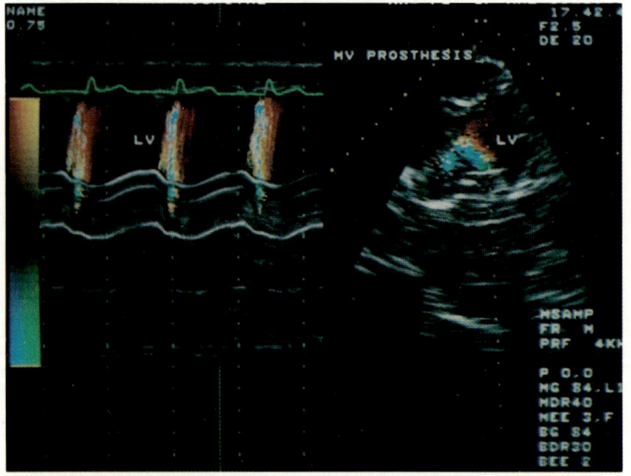

FIGURE 8-18—*Color Doppler of a prosthetic mitral valve. Color M-mode illustrates the aliasing and variance in the display of a normally functioning valve. LV = left ventricle.*

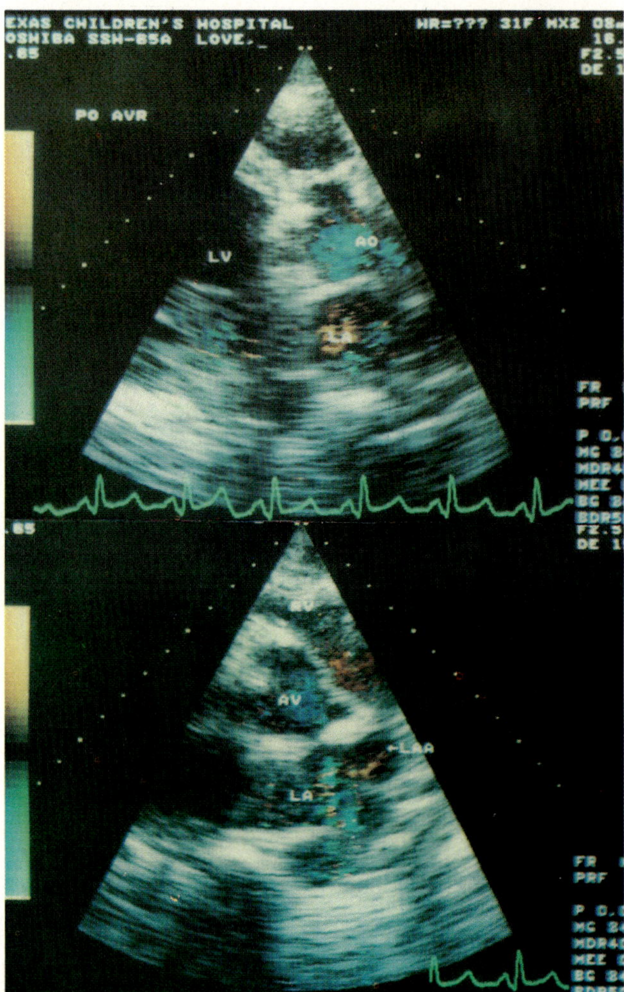

FIGURE 8-19—*Color Doppler of a prosthetic aortic valve (St. Jude) immediately after implantation. Note the eccentric direction of flow velocity in the ascending aorta (AO) in a parasternal scan (upper panel). The patient had moderately severe mitral insufficiency which is difficult to evaluate because of the prosthesis and posterior reverberations. Short-axis scans show variance and aliasing in the left atrium (LA) and left atrial appendage (LAA) (lower panel).*

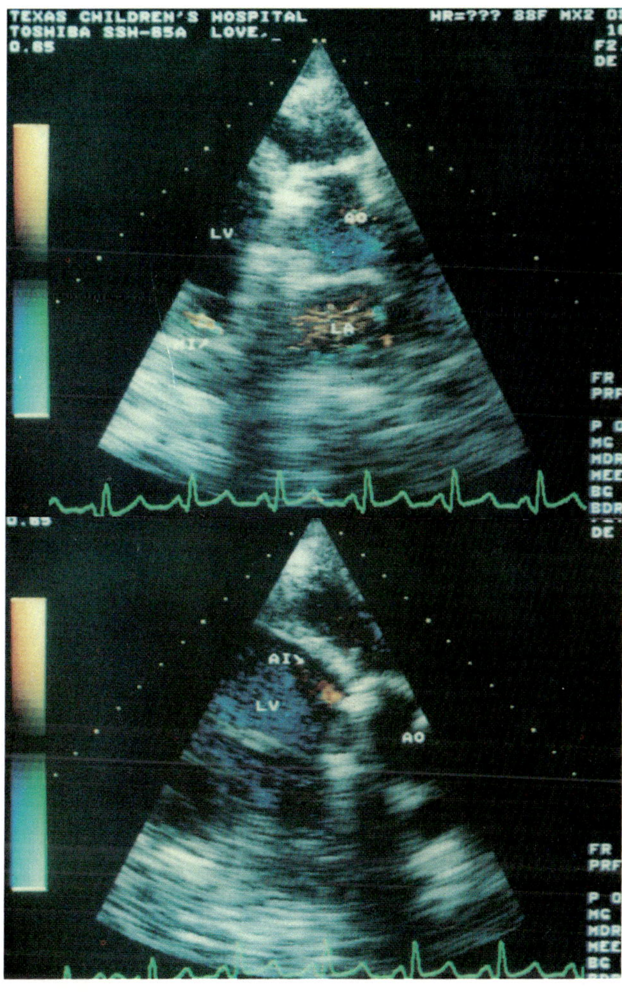

FIGURE 8-20—*Parasternal systolic (upper panel) and diastolic (lower panel) views of an aortic prosthesis. There is a normal amount of aortic insufficiency (AI) from the prosthetic valve (red jet in lower panel). AO = aorta; LA = left atrium; LV = left ventricle.*

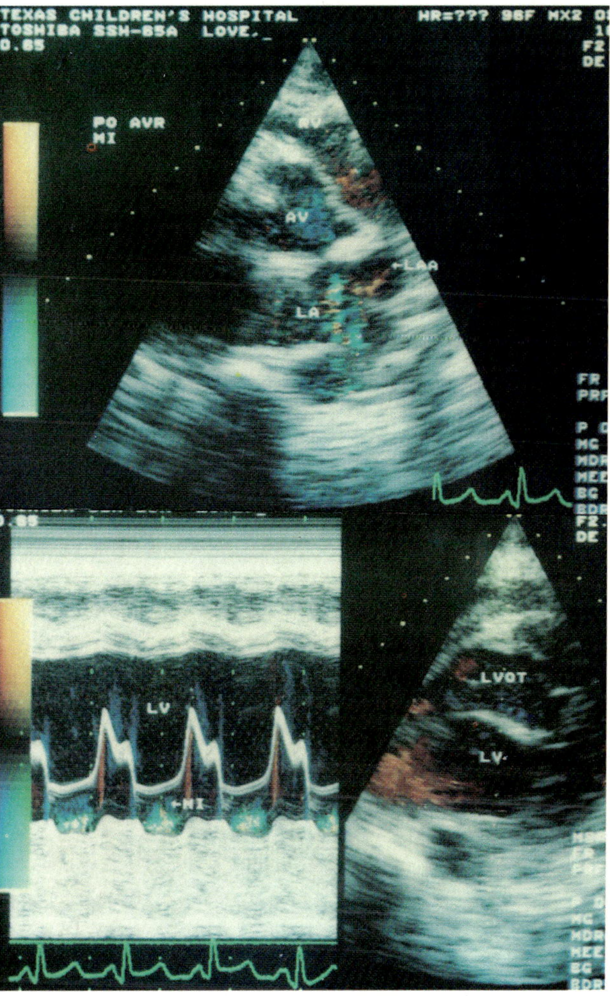

FIGURE 8-21—*Color Doppler of mitral insufficiency (MI) following aortic valve replacement. The color M-mode through the left ventricular outflow tract (LVOT) and left ventricle (LV) illustrates the timing of the regurgitation.*

References

1. Ortiz E, Robinson PJ, Dearfield JE, et al: Localization of ventricular septal defects by simultaneous display of superimposed colour Doppler and cross sectional echocardiographic images. Br Heart J 54: 53-60, 1985.
2. Ludomirsky A, Huhta JC, Vick GW, et al: Color Doppler detection of multiple ventricular septal defects. Circulation, 1986 (in press).
3. Colvin E, Nanda N, Bargeron LM: Color Doppler flow mapping in atrioventricular septal defects. Circulation 72(Suppl III):III- 436, 1985 (abstr).
4. Bommer WJ, Tam K, Ehret R, Rebeck, K: Two-dimensional real-time flow imaging of prosthetic heart valves. J Am Coll Cardiol 5:326, 1985.
5. Ciobanu M, Abbasi AS, Allen M: Pulsed Doppler echocardiography in the diagnosis and estimation of severity of aortic insufficiency. Am J Cardiol 49:339-343, 1982.
6. Byard CE, Perry GJ, Roitman DI, et al: Quantitative assessment of aortic regurgitation by color Doppler. Circulation 72(4):III-146, 1985 (abstr).
7. Hoit B, Howard DH, Sahn D, et al: Clinical studies of the efficacy of color flow mapping Doppler for evaluation of prosthetic heart valves. J Am Coll Cardiol 5:527, 1985.

Chapter 9

Cardiomyopathies and Coronary Arterial Abnormalities

David A. Danford, M.D.

Two-dimensional and M- mode echocardiography provide a wealth of anatomical and functional information in both dilated and hypertrophic cardiomyopathies. The addition of color Doppler can highlight some of the abnormal hemodynamics present in cardiomyopathies. Consequently, color Doppler is a potentially useful adjunct to previously established echocardiographic methods for evaluating these processes. As a complementary technique, color Doppler does not eliminate the need for high-quality two-dimensional and M-mode echocardiography in cardiomyopathy. As we shall see, it helps to focus the standard pulsed and continuous-wave Doppler examinations, but does not, at the present state of technology, supplant them.

Hypertrophic Cardiomyopathy

Color Doppler can detect any of several abnormal intracardiac flow patterns that may be present in hypertrophic cardiomyopathy.[1] For example, ejection of blood through a dynamic subaortic stenosis produces acceleration and turbulence which can be detected by color Doppler. With the transducer at the cardiac apex, the flow of blood away from the transducer is abnormally turbulent and may alias in late systole. Ejected blood may have to turn a relatively sharp corner between its original direction deep in the left ventricle and its final direction as it passes the subaortic obstruction (Figure 9-1). This passage results in turbulence and aliasing in the distal left ventricular outflow tract. Even from the parasternal transducer position, the predominant red-coded flow toward the transducer during systole is punctuated with blue coding for aliasing and substantial yellow-green coding for variance. This finding should prompt careful multiwindow continuous-wave Doppler examination of the left ventricular outflow tract for measurement of the maximal velocity.

Mitral valve insufficiency, a common hemodynamic problem in hypertrophic cardiomyopathy, may also be recognized in the parasternal or the apical view with systolic gating.[2-4] The mitral insufficiency jet goes away from the transducer at high velocity into the left atrium (Figure 9-1).

Abnormal ventricular filling occurs in hypertrophic cardiomyopathy with the potential for unusually oriented inflow patterns (Figure 9-2), perhaps due to distortion of papillary muscle and chordal support structures due to hypertrophy. Unusually prominent high- velocity aliasing patterns may be seen during late diastolic atrial-mediated left ventricular flilling in hypertrophic cardiomyopathy (Figure 9-2). Aliasing of ventricular late diastolic filling in the absence of early diastolic aliasing, or simply greater prominence of the late diastolic aliasing may be apparent by color Doppler. This finding should prompt careful pulsed Doppler examination of the left and right ventricular inflow for precise measurement of the E-wave and A-wave velocities.

Dilated Cardiomyopathy

Color Doppler may also detect the abnormal intracardiac hemodynamics present in dilated cardiomyopathy. As noted above in the discussion of hypertrophic cardiomyopathy, mitral valve insufficiency may be detected in dilated cardiomyopathy (Figure 9-3). In addition, tricuspid valve insufficiency may be apparent in dilated cardiomyopathy from the apical view or the parasternal short-axis view. When tricuspid valve insufficiency is severe, systemic venous flow reversal in the inferior vena cava or hepatic veins may be detected (see Chapter 4). For the same reasons why recording of normal prograde pulmonary venous flow is difficult (see Chapter 2), the detection of pulmonary venous flow reversal, which is no doubt present in severe mitral regurgitation

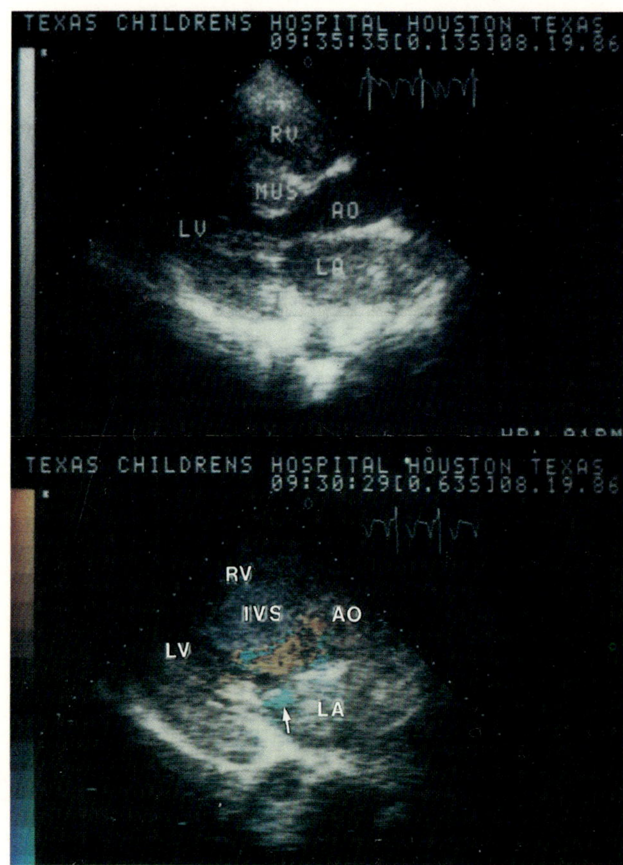

FIGURE 9-1—*With the transducer at the left sternal border and the plane of ultrasound oriented along the long axis of the left ventricle, the septal hypertrophy characteristic of hypertrophic obstructive cardiomyopathy is apparent (upper panel). Color Doppler in this view (lower panel) shows considerable frequency variance coding (yellow) injected into the red signal of left ventricular ejection along the septum into the proximal aorta. In addition, blue signal due to high-velocity flow is appreciated distal to the left ventricular outflow tract narrowing. The arrow indicates a green signal from mitral insufficiency. Ao = aorta; IVS = interventricular septum; LA = left atrium; LV = left ventricle; RV = right ventricle.*

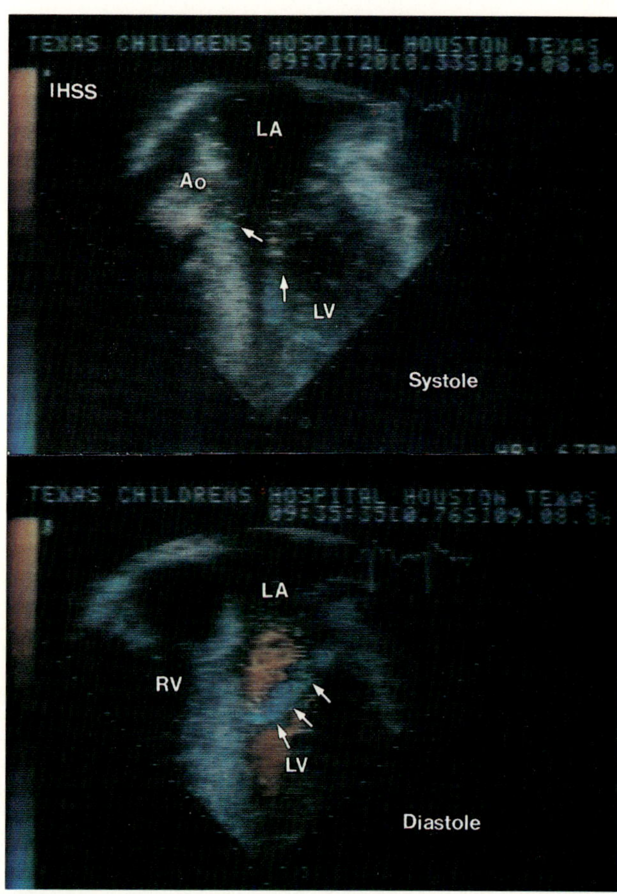

FIGURE 9-2—*An apical four-chamber view in systole (upper panel) in hypertrophic cardiomyopathy shows nonturbulent flow away from the transducer (blue) from the apex to the mid-ventricular level. Aliasing and turbulence are demonstrated in the distal left ventricular outflow tract. Note the apparent change in direction (arrows) between flows deep in the ventricle and those higher in the outflow tract. In late diastole (lower panel) with the transducer at the apex, the left ventricular inflow pattern in hypertrophic cardiomyopathy is shown. The flow is generally toward the transducer (red); however, an unusual aliasing pattern is present, suggesting that the fastest ventricular inflow (blue) is not directed apically so much as it is toward the ventricular septum. Alterations in mitral valve support structures by the severe and asymmetrical ventricular hypertrophy may be responsible for this abnormal filling pattern. The unusual degree of aliasing during atrial-mediated late diastolic filling may provide a clue that ventricular compliance is abnormal. A careful pulsed Doppler recording of left ventricular inflow should confirm this. Ao = aorta; LA = left atrium; LV = left ventricle; RV = right ventricle.*

due to cardiomyopathy, stretches beyond the limitations of the present technology. Technical advances may soon make this flow detectable and it may prove useful in grading severity of mitral regurgitation.

Less commonly, semilunar valve insufficiency may be apparent by color Doppler in dilated cardiomyopathy. Pulmonary valve insufficiency in dilated cardiomyopathy can be demonstrated as a diastolic high-velocity jet coming toward the transducer in the parasternal or subcostal position using a sufficiently sensitive system (see Chapter 4).

Ventricular inflow blood flow velocity patterns in dilated cardiomyopathy may be abnormal. Figure 9-4 demonstrates diastolic swirling of blood within a dilated left ventricle in mid-diastole. Note the multidirectional low-velocity currents within the left ventricle giving a "tiger-stripe" appearance.

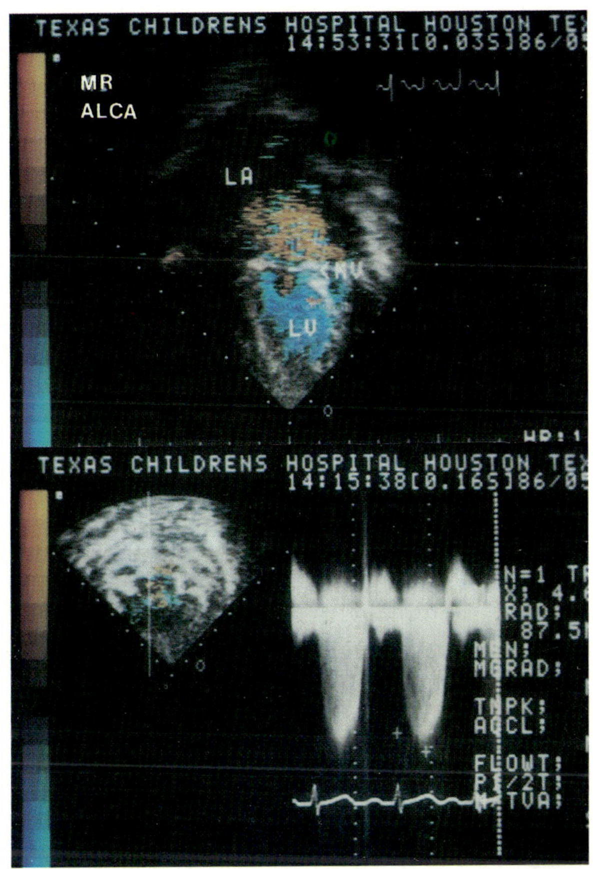

FIGURE 9-3—*Anomalous left coronary artery and left ventricular dysfunction. From the cardiac apex, the plane of ultrasound is oriented in the standard four-chamber view. Color Doppler (upper panel) shows a strong broad red signal with variance in the left atrium during systole. Continuous-wave Doppler interrogation (lower panel) demonstrates that this is a high-velocity flow directed away from the transducer. The predominantly red color is due to aliasing. ALCA = anomalous left coronary artery; LA = left atrium; LV = left ventricle; MR = mitral regurgitation; MV = mitral valve.*

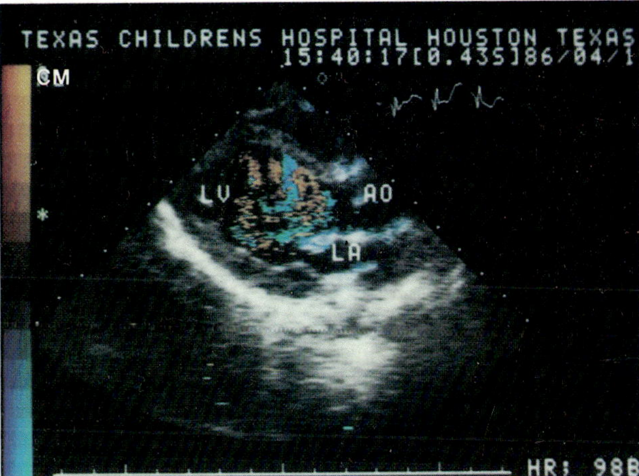

FIGURE 9-4—*This diastolic frame from a patient with dilated cardiomyopathy is taken with the transducer at the left sternal border and the ultrasound plane directed along the long axis of the left ventricle. A distinct swirling of flow signals (red and blue) is seen after the completion of rapid filling. AO = aorta; CM = cardiomyopathy; LA = left atrium; LV = left ventricle.*

Coronary Arterial Abnormalities

The presentation of any infant with an unexplained dilated cardiomyopathy should raise the question of a coronary arterial anomaly, particularly anomalous origin of the left coronary artery from the pulmonary artery. Patients with anomalous origin of the left coronary artery from the pulmonary artery will show many of the features of dilated cardiomyopathy outlined above, and in addition may have a characteristic color Doppler finding in the main pulmonary artery. Figure 9-5 shows a jet of blood entering the main pulmonary artery during diastole from the mouth of the anomalous left coronary artery. This is a useful positive finding when it is present; however, the absence of this color Doppler finding does not exclude the possibility of anomalous left coronary artery. For example, patients in whom the pulmonary vascular resistance is high may not exhibit detectable jetting of blood into the pulmonary artery. Also, the occasional patient with anomalous origin of the left coronary artery from a distal pulmonary artery may not show the characteristic diastolic flow pattern in the main pulmonary artery illustrated in Figure 9- 4. Nevertheless, many patients with anomalous left coronary artery can be detected with color Doppler. Appropriate further evaluation of this abnormal color flow pattern would be the assessment of severity of mitral insufficiency by measurement of the left atrial size using two-dimensional and/or M-mode measurements and by area mapping of the regurgitant jet in the left atrium (see Chapter 4) confirmed by careful pulsed Doppler mapping within the left atrium.

Other coronary arterial abnormalities may be detected using color Doppler. For example, a coronary artery fistula may be detected by the appearance of continuous turbulent flow within an enlarged coronary artery. It is often possible to trace the course of the fistula to its point of drainage using multiple imaging planes and diastolic gating. Figures 9-6 and 9-7 demonstrate the path of a left coronary artery to right ventricular apex fistula. The proximal portions of this fistula are well demonstrated in the parasternal short-axis and short-axis oblique views (Figure 9-6), while the distal portions are well demonstrated in the apical views (Figure 9-7). Very small fistulae with small volume of blood flow may be

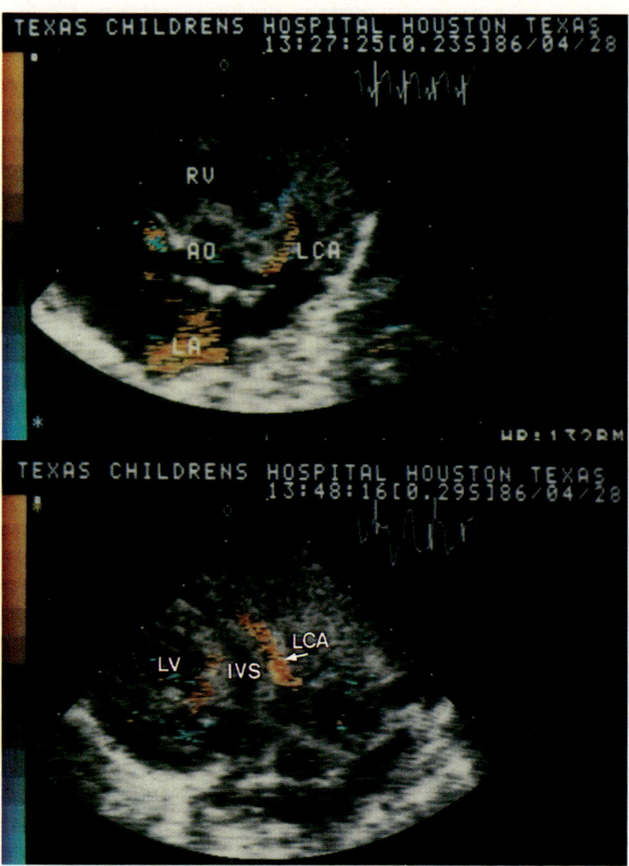

FIGURE 9-6—*Left coronary artery fistula (three weeks old). Upper panel: a diastolic gated flow map is shown with the transducer in the parasternal short-axis orientation. Note the prominent red-yellow signal originating from turbulent blood flow in the proximal left coronary artery (LCA). Angulation of the transducer that produces an oblique short axis somewhat lower in the heart (lower panel) demonstrates continuation of this coronary flow along the upper portion of the interventricular septum. Ao = aorta; IVS = interventricular septum; LA = left atrium; LV = left ventricle; RV = right ventricle.*

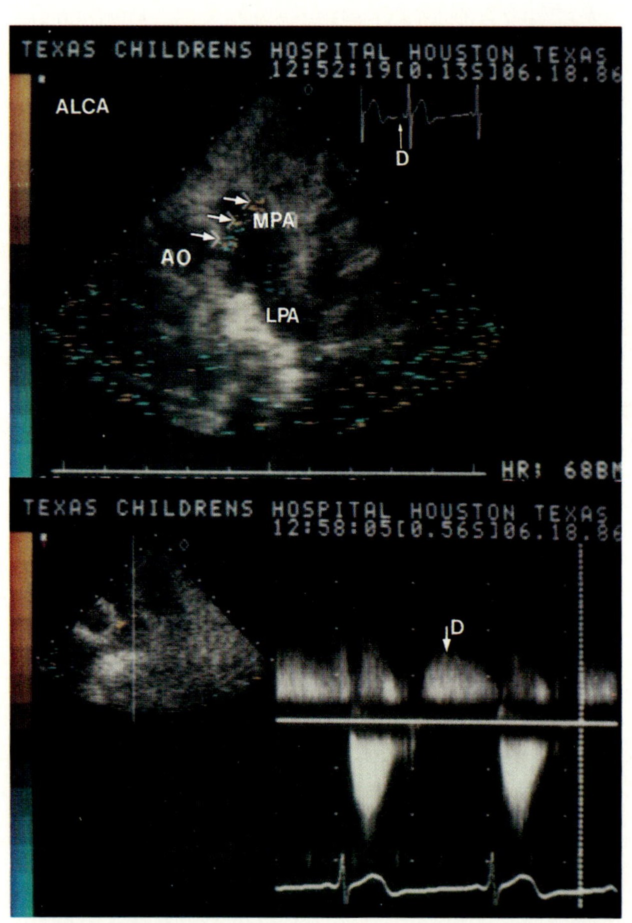

FIGURE 9-5—*With the transducer very high on the left sternal border and the plane of ultrasound oriented across the short axis of the ascending aorta, a gated diastolic (D) frame is shown in this infant with anomalous left coronary artery (ALCA) from the main pulmonary artery (upper panel). Note the linear jet (arrows) indicating turbulent blood flow entering the main pulmonary artery. Continuous-wave Doppler (lower panel) confirms this abnormal flow pattern reminiscent of patent ductus arteriosus. The orientation of the jet entering the pulmonary artery effectively excludes patent ductus arteriosus. Ao = aorta; LPA = left pulmonary artery; MPA = main pulmonary artery.*

difficult or impossible to detect with some current color Doppler systems.

Normal coronary arterial blood flow is generally not detectable with current color Doppler technology. Substantial improvement of presently available color Doppler systems will be required in order to allow detection of normal coronary arterial blood flow and to distinguish it from abnormal coronary arterial flow to ischemic myocardium. Application of color Doppler to coronary flow problems in Kawasaki disease therefore awaits substantial technological advances. The more gross findings of dilated cardiomyopathy that occasionally occur in Kawasaki disease (valvular insufficiency, inflow swirling) are, however, potentially detectable by color Doppler now.

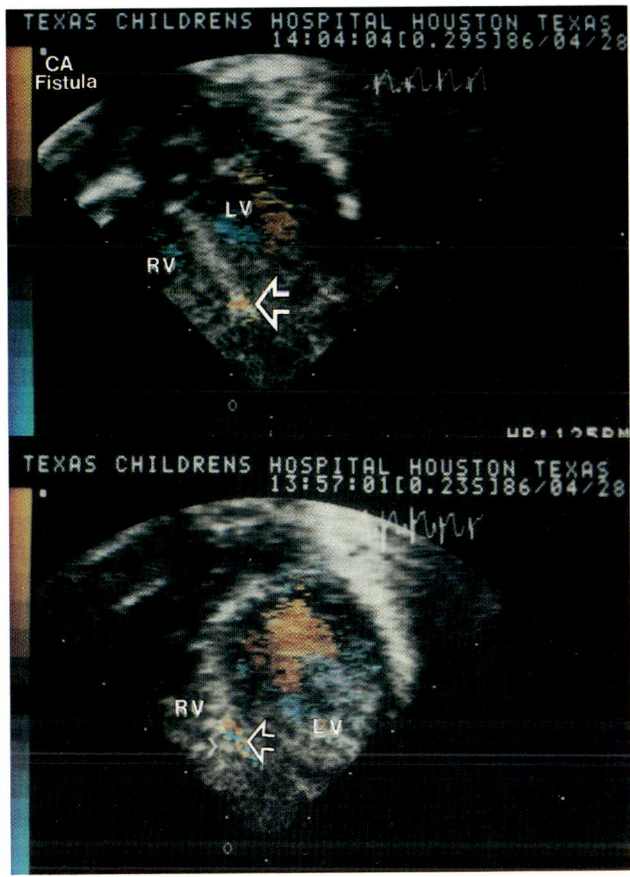

FIGURE 9-7—*The coronary artery fistula (same patient as in Figure 9-6) is seen with the transducer at the cardiac apex angled slightly anterior to the standard four-chamber view (upper panel). The lower panel shows the fistula in a more posterior four-chamber view. Ao = aorta; LV = left ventricle; RV = right ventricle; arrows indicate the coronary artery fistula.*

References

1. Nishimura RA, Tajik AJ, Reeder GS, Seward JB: Evaluation of hypertrophic cardiomyopathy by Doppler color flow imaging: Initial observations. Mayo Clin Proc 61:631-639, 1986.
2. Miyatake K, Izumi S, Okamoto M, et al: Semiquantitative grading of severity of mitral regurgitation by real-time two-dimensional Doppler flow imaging technique. J Am Coll Cardiol 7:82-88, 1986.
3. Saenz CB, Deumite J, Roitman DI, et al: Limitations of color Doppler in quantitative assessment of mitral regurgitation. Circulation 72(Suppl III):III-99, 1985 (abstr).
4. Chandraratna PAN, Minagoe S, Wade M, et al: Demonstration of regurgitant stream shape and direction in mitral and tricuspid regurgitation by two-dimensional Doppler color flow mapping. J Am Coll Cardiol 5:454, 1985.

Chapter 10

Aorta and Veins

James C. Huhta, M.D.

Color Doppler in the Evaluation of the Aorta

The aorta has four distinct parts that require a segmental approach to imaging[1] and Doppler evaluation[2,3]: (1) the ascending aorta, (2) the aortic arch, (3) the aortic isthmus and upper descending aorta, and (4) the lower descending aorta. Color Doppler evaluation of the aorta in areas where it is changing direction may be confusing because the direction coding changes and some of the velocities in the aorta are beyond the point of aliasing using the equipment available today. Parallel alignment with the ascending aorta, for example, requires that the transducer be placed either in the suprasternal notch or in the apical or subcostal regions, and all of these echocardiographic windows place the sampling site of interest at least 6 centimeters away from the transducer. Increased distance also demands a high sensitivity for the detection of blood flow. Therefore, in adults or older children with congenital abnormalities of the aorta, color Doppler may be impractical or add little to the usual two-dimensional/pulsed and continuous-wave Doppler examination. However, color Doppler may be of use as an aid to assessing the severity of a lesion that causes diastolic reversal in the aorta, such as aortic insufficiency (see Chapter 4) or patent ductus arteriosus (see Chapter 5).

Ascending Aorta

Systolic jets of high intensity in the ascending aorta such as those in aortic stenosis (see Chapter 3), may be visualized from the suprasternal or high parasternal approaches (Figures 10-1 and 10-2). Color Doppler may be useful for alignment with the jet direction for quantitation of the peak instantaneous pressure gradient. One unknown in this estimation is the third angle or azimuthal plane. Color Doppler adds a second dimension to the visualization of aortic stenosis jets but such flow disturbances are three-dimensional and two-dimensional flow imaging may lead to a false sense of security in pressure gradient estimation. As always, the peak jet velocity should be recorded using an optimized transducer without imaging from suprasternal, parasternal, apical, and subcostal positions.[4] Jet localization is improved using two color Doppler imaging planes.

Aortopulmonary communications such as origin of a pulmonary artery from the ascending aorta or aortopulmonary window[5,6] can be difficult to diagnose with imaging alone owing to echo dropout between these structures. By combining color Doppler and imaging, these types of errors should be avoided but a high index of suspicion is necessary to make the diagnosis.

Marfan's disease causes dilation of the aortic sinuses and ascending aorta, and is associated with dissection of the aorta and aortic insufficiency. The dilation of the aorta is associated with turbulent systolic flow in the ascending aorta. The distribution of velocities in the aorta may be important in following the course of the disease in combination with careful monitoring of the size of the structures.

Aortic Arch

Congenital aortic arch abnormalities require high-resolution imaging for diagnosis and associated hemodynamic abnormalities can usually be inferred.[7] Color Doppler evaluation combined with imaging has the advantage of screening for abnormal velocities in the arch and its branches. The aortic arch often contains systolic velocities that result in aliasing from suprasternal notch color Doppler (Figure 10-3). The brachiocephalic branches of the aorta are sites of an increase in velocity and even under normal circumstances of resting cardiac output and pressures, aliasing may occur at these sites (Figure 10-4), particularly in infants and neonates. Color Doppler is most useful in detecting the cause of a contin-

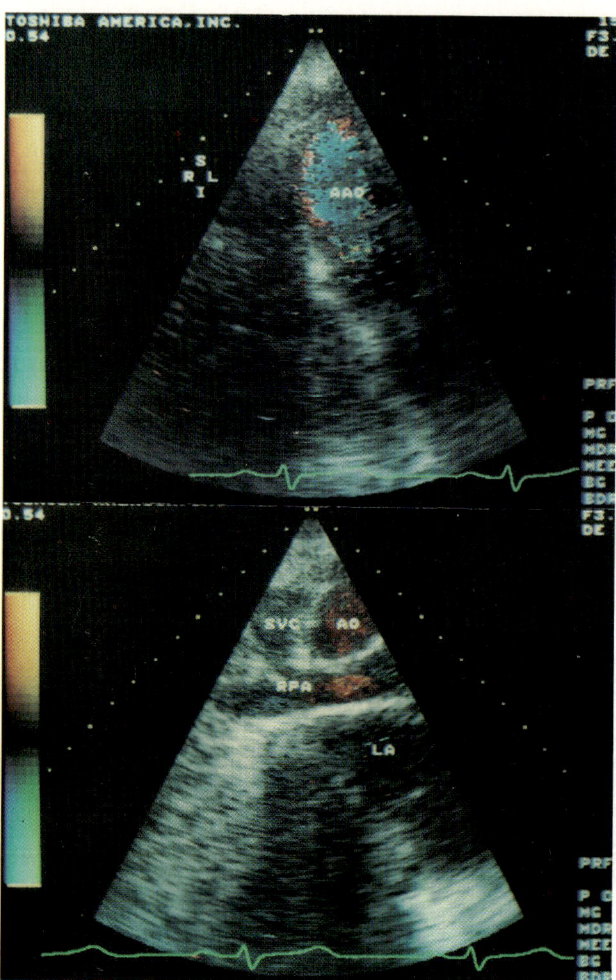

FIGURE 10-1—*Suprasternal systolic frames of the ascending aorta (AAO) from coronal (upper panel) and slightly more posterior projections (lower panel). Aliasing in the ascending aorta (blue flow toward the transducer superiorly) is present except near the aortic walls. The aorta (Ao) is seen in cross-section at the level of the transverse arch with the right pulmonary artery (RPA) inferior to it. The right superior vena cava is to the right of the aorta (SVC) and the left atrium (LA) is inferior. I = inferior; L = left; R = right; S = superior.*

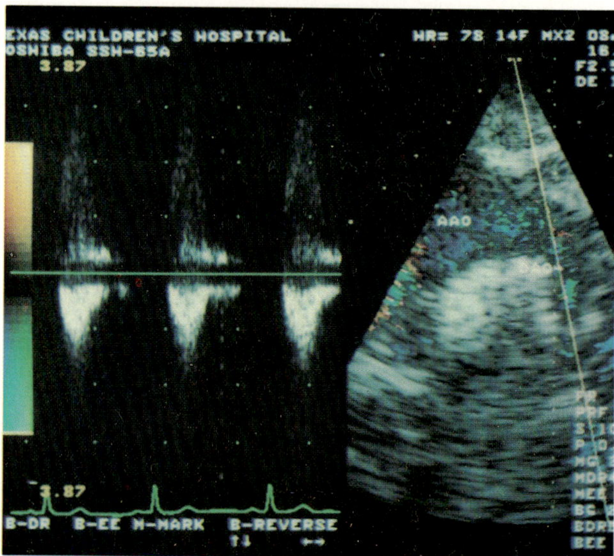

FIGURE 10-2—*Suprasternal color Doppler-directed pulsed Doppler sampling in the descending aorta with aliasing at the aortic isthmus. AAO = ascending aorta.*

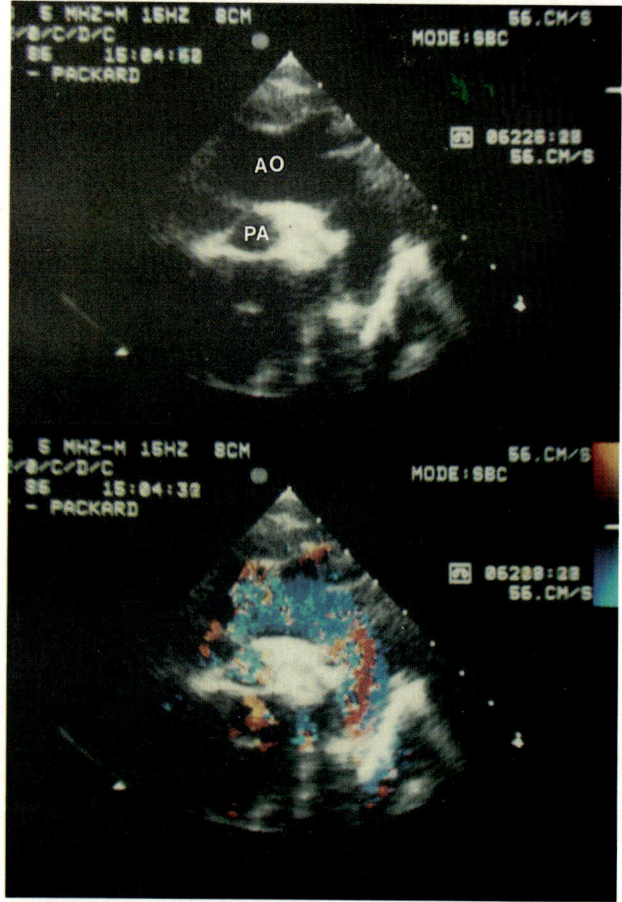

FIGURE 10-3—*Two-dimensional imaging (upper panel) and color Doppler (lower panel) in the aorta (AO) with color aliasing plus variance in the upper descending aorta and in the ductal diverticulum. PA = pulmonary artery.*

uous murmur such as an arteriovenous fistula from one of these arteries or abnormal runoff as seen in coarctation of the aorta with collateral arteries. The application to the assessment of systemic-to- pulmonary shunts is discussed in Chapter 8.

Anomalous origin of the right subclavian artery is common and the diagnosis can be inferred by scanning of the right innominate artery and its normal right carotid and right subclavian branches.[1] Color Doppler is potentially more sensitive than imaging alone in the recognition of this artery and its retroesophageal course.

The diagnosis of *double aortic arch* is made easier

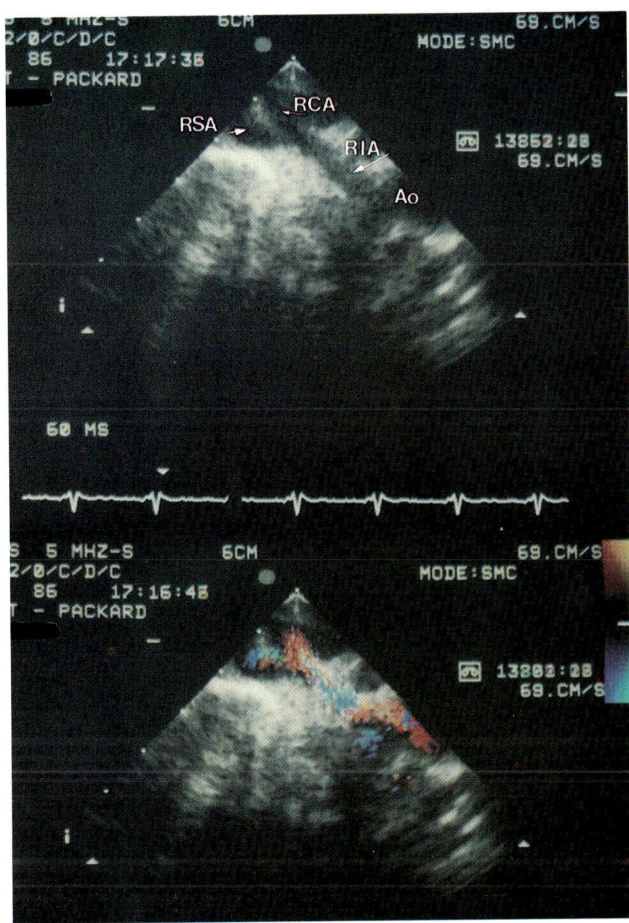

FIGURE 10-4—*Suprasternal scanning toward the right shoulder showing the right innominate artery (RIA) and its right carotid (RCA) and right subclavian (RSA) branches. Note the presence of dispersion or variance as indicated by the mosaic pattern on color Doppler (lower panel). Ao = aorta.*

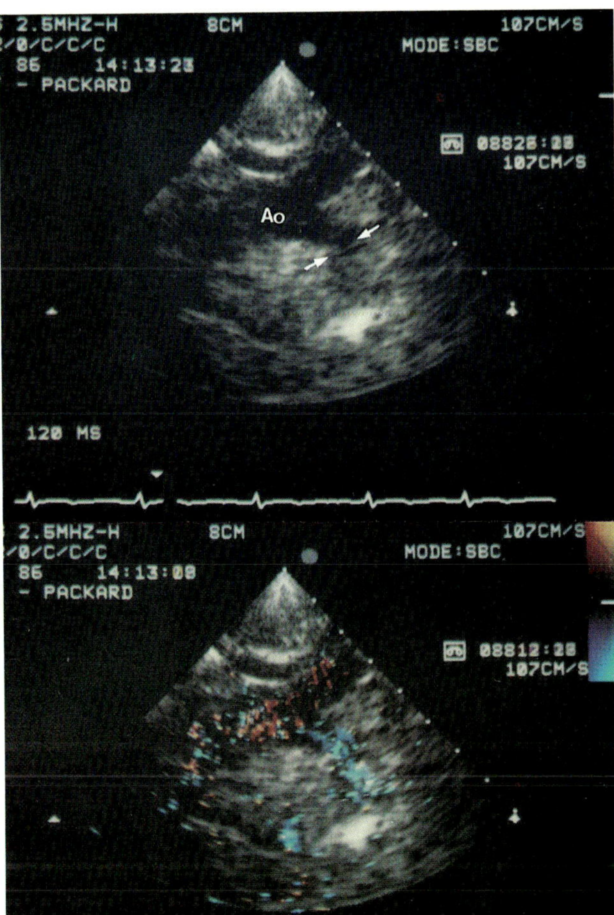

FIGURE 10-5—*Suprasternal scan of the aortic arch (Ao) in coarctation of the aorta. There is aliasing and variance in the color display in the aortic isthmus (arrows).*

with color Doppler because both arches can be recognized and traced, and the presence of an associated patent ductus arteriosus can be diagnosed.

Arteriovenous malformation in the head (vein of Galen aneurysm) in the neonate presents with congestive heart failure with nonspecific signs on two-dimensional imaging such as cardiac dilation, superior caval and carotid artery dilation, and right- to-left ductal shunting. The large increase in blood returning to the right atrium gives a dramatic appearance on color Doppler similar to the findings in total anomalous pulmonary venous connection (see below).

Aortic Isthmus and Upper Descending Aorta

Color Doppler can give insight into the hemodynamics of congenital lesions causing obstruction of the aorta. In *coarctation of the aorta*, the site of obstruction may be difficult to visualize (Figure 10-5). In coarctation of the aorta in infancy, pulsed Doppler has shown left-to-right shunting of the ductus arteriosus in some neonates. This shunting from the upper descending aorta above the coarctation to the pulmonary artery may be a significant cause of increased left-to-right shunt. This shunt is in close proximity to the systolic right-to-left ductal shunting to the descending aorta and the coarctation jet from upper to lower aorta. Color Doppler has the advantage that it can separate two such jets occurring close together.

Blood flow velocity increases proximal to the site of coarctation and the jet can sometimes be seen below it. If there is no antegrade flow across the coarctation, as in some older children and adults, Doppler can be useful in detecting this and in selecting patients for balloon angioplasty of the coarctation, which is possible only if there is patency. The result of angioplasty can be evalu-

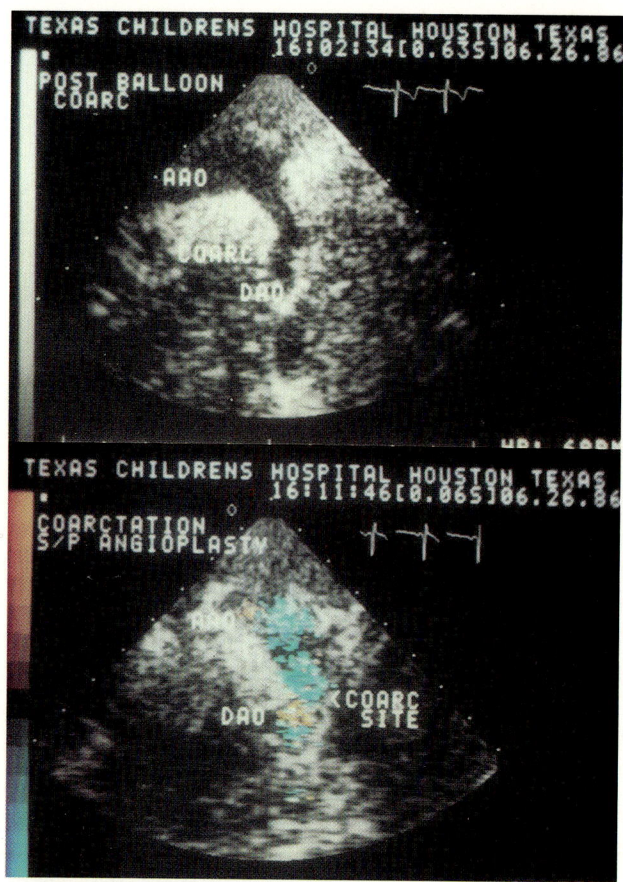

FIGURE 10-6—*Imaging and color Doppler assessment of the site of coarctation following balloon angioplasty. AAO = ascending aorta; DAO = descending aorta.*

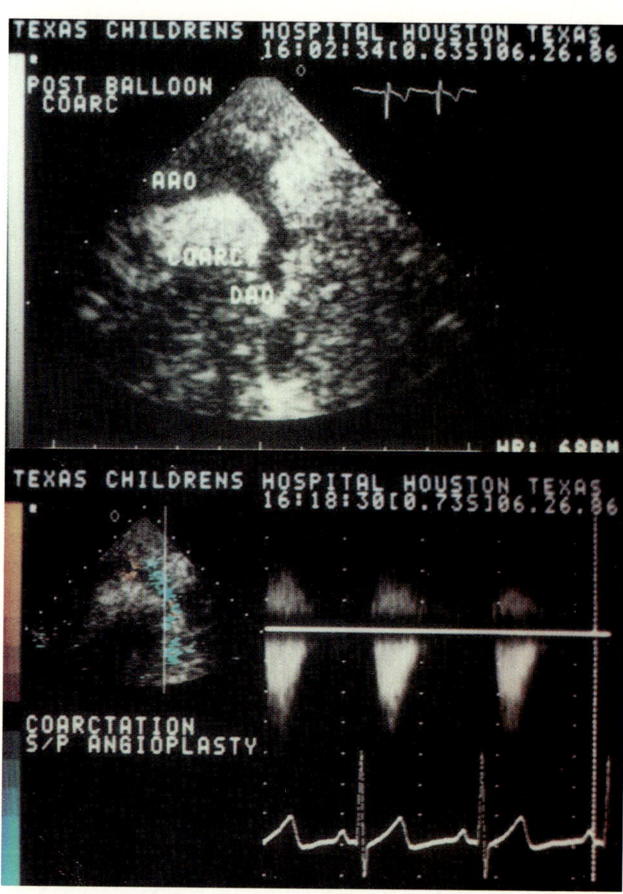

FIGURE 10-7—*Imaging and continuous-wave Doppler assessment of coarctation after angioplasty showing a maximum systolic velocity of 1.7 meters per second.*

ated by color and continuous-wave Doppler (Figures 10-6 and 10-7).

Flow reversal in the descending aorta is a well-recognized sign of significant *aortic insufficiency* or large left-to-right shunt from an *aortopulmonary communication*. Normally, there is slight forward flow at the aortic isthmus in diastole and any flow reversal detected by color Doppler with suprasternal notch imaging of the aorta is abnormal (see Chapter 4).

Abdominal Aorta

The normal flow pattern in the abdominal aorta is similar to that described above and, because the impedance of the lower body is low, there is normally diastolic runoff in all parts of the descending aorta toward the distal arterial bed (see Chapter 2). The abdominal aorta can be difficult to image because of bowel air, but the origin of the celiac and superior mesenteric arteries can usually be imaged in sagittal scans from the subcostal region. The angle of incidence of the ultrasound with the descending aorta is optimal for imaging but the Doppler sampling and color Doppler are hampered by an angle of nearly 90 degrees. As a result, the systolic flow may appear red or blue or both, depending on the angulation.

Systemic Veins

A segmental approach to the systemic veins includes evaluation of the superior vena cava, the inferior vena cava, the coronary sinus, the hepatic veins and their connections, and the other possible sites of abnormality such as a persistent left superior vena cava. Color Doppler may not detect the normal flow in these regions unless the sensitivity of the sampling regarding intensity and velocity is sufficiently high. A low-velocity signal may be intense owing to a large flow in a venous structure, but the Doppler shift at that depth may be below the threshold for display. Therefore, it is important to know the cut-off frequency of the filtering in a particular color Doppler display. In parts of the circulation where low-velocity, large-volume flows occur, the use of intensity color Doppler mapping or a power density mode has improved the ability to visualize blood flow. Because the display is the intensity of flow, once it is detected with a direction coding, the display is relatively insensitive to the angle of incidence of the ultrasound beam. For example, imaging perpendicular to a vessel during continuous flow will show an uninterrupted display of flow changing abruptly in direction code perpendicular to flow.

Superior vena caval flow can be visualized by suprasternal or subcostal scans. In the latter, the superior caval blood flow velocity is directed toward the transducer, or red (Figure 10-8). Superior caval obstruction is manifested by a loss of pulsatility in the blood flow velocity and there may be a jet of greater than 1.5 meters per second across such an area by pulsed or continuous-wave Doppler. Color Doppler may be normal (see Chapter 2), or show quite dramatic findings of obstruction but should not be used exclusively to exclude obstruction because of the dependence of flow velocity on the volume of flow across the obstruction and the very high compliance of the systemic venous system.

The *inferior vena cava* and hepatic venous branches can be imaged without difficulty, and their size, and the pattern of flow velocity in it, can be very useful in estimating the venous pressure and diagnosing disturbances such as tricuspid insufficiency. For example, reversal of flow in the hepatic veins (Figure 10-9) can be due to obstruction to right atrial outflow or to elevated atrial pressure from valve regurgitation.

Persistent left superior vena cava can be diagnosed accurately with two-dimensional imaging,[8] but color Doppler is useful if the differential is between this diagnosis and anomalous pulmonary venous connection to this structure with flow in a superior direction (see below). Flow abnormalities of the coronary sinus result in dilation of this structure, usually from drainage of a persistent left superior vena cava. Coronary artery fistula to the coronary sinus will cause a large coronary sinus and a prominent color Doppler appearance of increased flow.

Azygos continuation of the inferior vena cava can be diagnosed by its position posterior and lateral with respect to the spine and its retrocardiac course as it ascends either on the left or the right to connect with the ipsilateral superior vena cava. The direction of flow in this structure can be confirmed by pulsed Doppler and by color Doppler by angling the transducer superior from a subcostal sagittal plane. The site of superior caval connection in these patients is usually to the top of the atrium with left atrial isomerism and the pattern of flow velocity in this region may aid in this diagnosis.

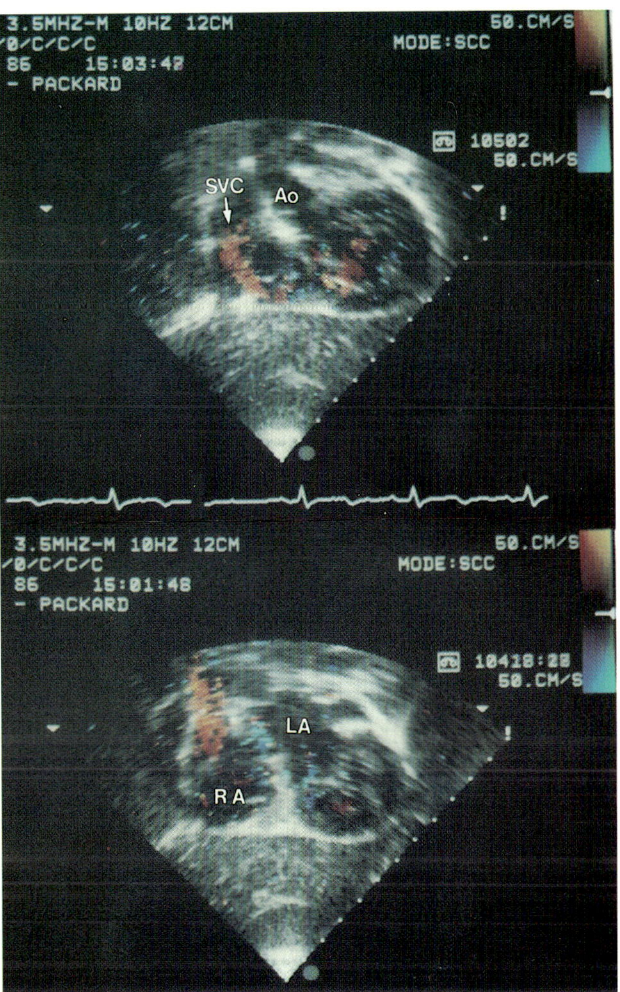

FIGURE 10-8—*Subcostal imaging plus color Doppler of the flow velocity from the superior vena cava (SVC) into the right atrium (RA) coded as red. Ao = aorta; LA = left atrium.*

Pulmonary Veins

Pulmonary venous connection to the left atrium via four pulmonary veins is a low-velocity circulation and is situated relatively far from Doppler sampling (see Chapter 2). Abnormalities of pulmonary venous flow velocity reflect either increased flow (as with atrial or ventricular septal defect) or pulmonary venous obstruction. Color Doppler is useful to direct pulsed or continuous-wave Doppler sampling when an abnormality is suspected. There is progressive acceleration of blood flow from the posterior left atrium to the mitral valve orifice as the four individual flows merge. Continuous-wave or pulsed Doppler sampling from the apex window yields the maximum velocities when obstruction to the left ventricular inflow is present.[9] However, the most common abnormality of the pulmonary veins is abnormal connection, either partial or total.

Partial Anomalous Pulmonary Venous Connection

Limited experience is available using color Doppler for the diagnosis of partial anomalous pulmonary venous connection, but the combination of imaging and color Doppler is superior to either alone. The most common site of partial connection is with a sinus venosus atrial septal defect and connection of the right upper pulmonary vein to the right superior vena cava. Color Doppler may be useful in defining the interconnection of pulmonary confluences, a difficult problem by any technique today.[10]

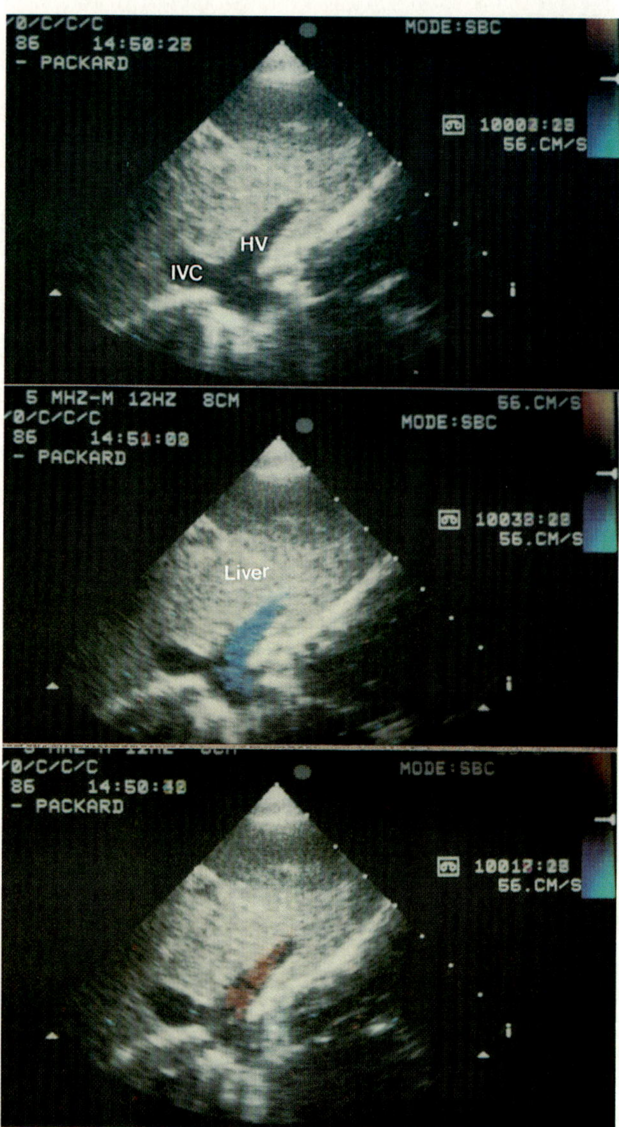

FIGURE 10-9—*Imaging and color Doppler (two lower panels) of the inferior vena cava (IVC) and the hepatic veins (HV) showing reversal of flow (red in lower panel) in the hepatic veins in this patient with tricupid insufficiency.*

Total Anomalous Pulmonary Venous Connection

The patterns of venous flow demonstrated by color flow mapping in patients with total anomalous pulmonary venous connection (TAPVC) depend on the location of pulmonary venous drainage.[10,11] In a patient with unobstructed *supracardiac* TAPVC, an increased volume of blood flow returns to the right atrium, causing dramatic color Doppler findings (Figure 10-10). With

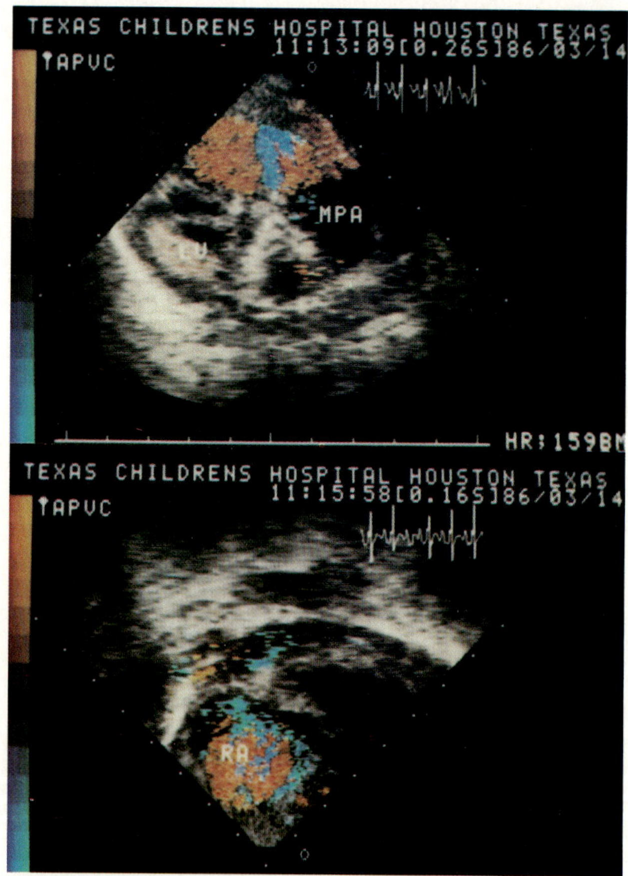

FIGURE 10-10—*Parasternal (upper panel) and apical (lower panel) views of an infant with total anomalous pulmonary venous connection (TAPVC) with the easily recognizable finding of prominent, turbulent flow in the right heart (RV in upper and RA in lower panel respectively). MPA = main pulmonary artery.*

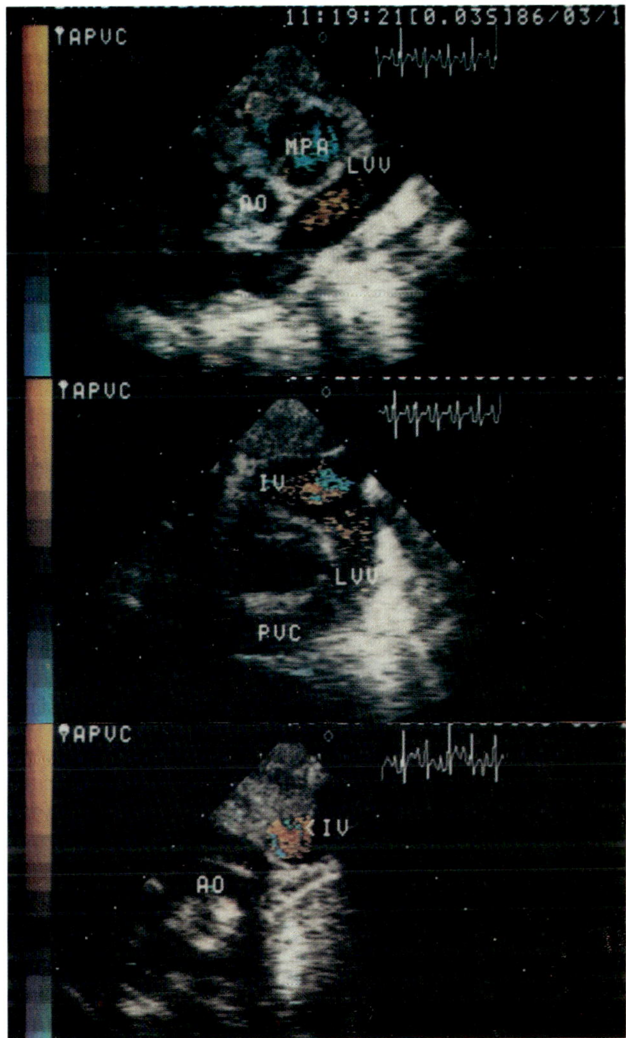

FIGURE 10-11—*Total anomalous pulmonary venous connection (TAPVC) to a left vertical vein (LVV) with drainage to the innominate vein (IV) and right atrium. Sequential scans of the pulmonary venous confluence (PVC) and the course of anomalous flow are obtained from high parasternal and suprasternal scans. AO = aorta; MPA = main pulmonary artery.*

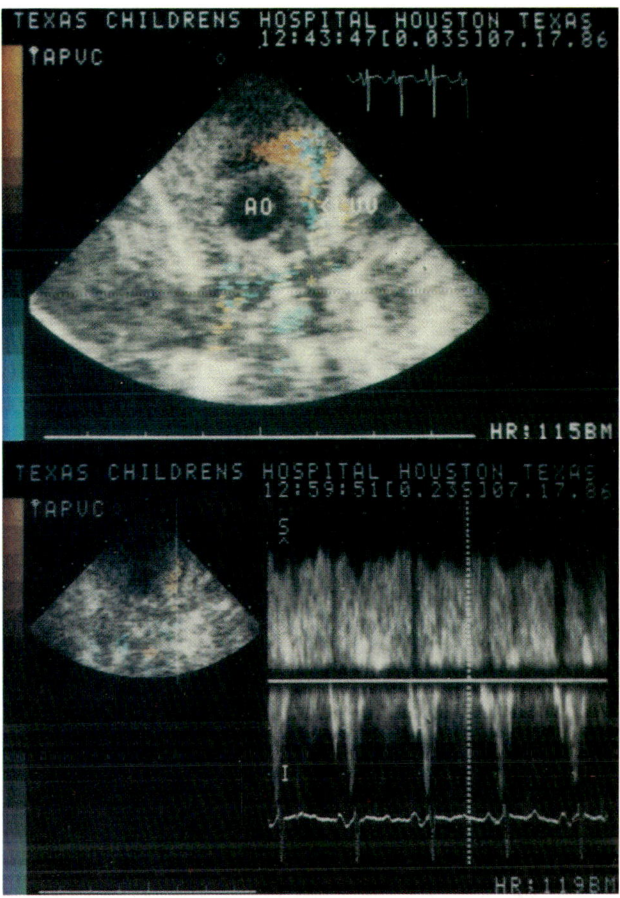

FIGURE 10-12—*Suprasternal continuous-wave Doppler of TAPVC to a left vertical vein (LVV) with a peak velocity of 1.5 meters per second guided by color Doppler. AO = aorta; I = inferior; S = superior.*

drainage to a left vertical vein, flow will be noted in the left vertical vein toward the transducer from the suprasternal notch (Figure 10-11). Increased velocities will be demonstrated in the left vertical vein, as well as the superior vena cava (Figure 10-12). In patients with pulmonary venous drainage to the coronary sinus, flow will be normal in the innominate vein and the superior vena cava, whereas drainage of the pulmonary veins to the right superior vena cava will be associated with increased flow patterns detectable at the site of insertion of the pulmonary veins into the SVC (Figure 10-13), although right superior caval dilation is present in TAPVC to a left vertical vein as well. Careful flow mapping, therefore, allows detection of the site of pulmonary venous drainage.

Infracardiac connection of the pulmonary veins occurs to the hepatic vein, portal vein, or inferior vena cava. In such cases flow in the inferior vena cava is increased and frequently there is flow disturbance. In addition, careful color Doppler of the vascular structures in the abdomen and the liver will detect the presence of the descending common pulmonary vein with flow directed caudally. As with supracardiac TAPVC, the precise location of pulmonary venous drainage can be detected by color flow mapping. In TAPVC, flow across the atrial septal defect occurs exclusively from right to left. The presence of left-to- right flow across the atrial septum excludes the diagnosis of TAPVC. As with other lesions associated with right-sided volume overload, TAPVC produces increased velocities across the tricuspid and pulmonary valves. These increases in flow are detectable using color Doppler. Finally, newborn infants with TAPVC and a patent ductus arteriosus frequently have bidirectional shunting at the ductal level which is demonstrable using color Doppler.

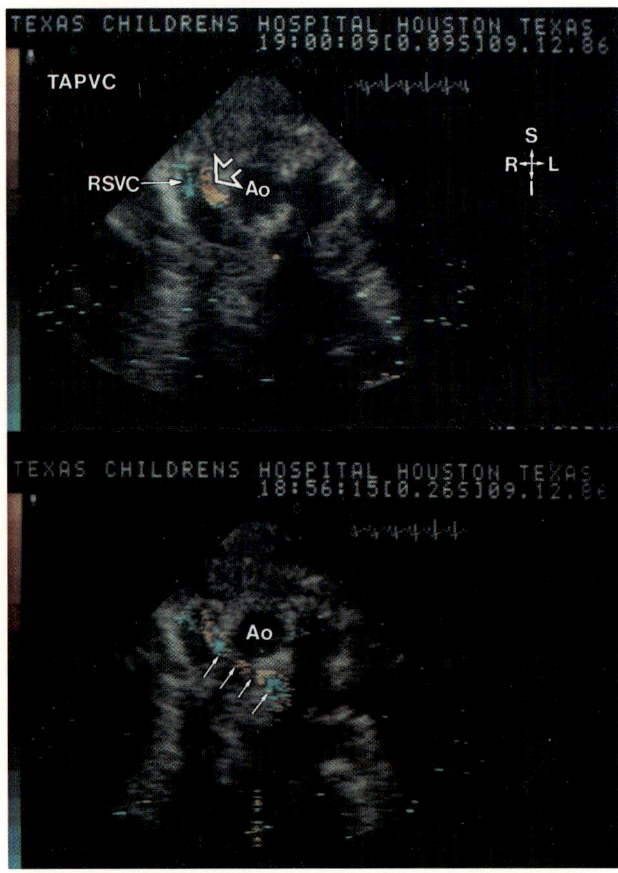

FIGURE 10-13—*Total anomalous pulmonary venous connection to the right superior vena cava (RSVC) on suprasternal scans. Note the normal inferior (blue) velocity simultaneous with the aliased jet at the site of connection (white arrow in upper panel). The pulmonary confluence communicated with the RSVC by a communicating vein behind the pulmonary artery (small arrows). I = inferior; L = left; R = right, S = superior.*

References

1. Huhta JC, Gutgesell HP, Latson LA, Huffines FD: Two-dimensional echocardiographic assessment of the aorta in infants and children with congenital heart disease. Circulation 70:417- 424, 1984.
2. Marx, GR, Allen HD: Accuracy and pitfalls of Doppler evaluation of the pressure gradient in aortic coaractation. J Am Coll Cardiol 7:1379-1385, 1986.
3. Hatle L: Assessment of aortic blood flow velocites with continuous wave Doppler ultrasound in the neonate and young child. J Am Coll Cardiol 5:113S-119S, 1985.
4. Currie PJ, Seward JB, Chan KL, et al: Continuous wave Doppler determination of right ventricular pressure: A simultaneous Doppler-catheterization study in 127 patients. J Am Coll Cardiol 6:750-756, 1985.
5. King D, Huhta JC, Gutgesell HP, Ott DA: Two-dimensional echocardiographic diagnosis of anomalous origin of the right pulmonary artery from the aorta: Differentiation from aortopulmonary window. J Am Coll Cardiol 4:351-355, 1984.
6. Smallhorn JF, Anderson RH, Macartney FJ: Two-dimensional echocardiographic assessment of communications between ascending aorta and pulmonary trunk or individual pulmonary arteries. Br Heart J 47:229-235, 1982.
7. Huhta JC: Pediatric Imaging/Doppler Ultrasound of the Chest: Extracardiac Diagnosis. Philadelphia, Lea & Febiger, 1986 (in press), Chap 5, Aortic Arch.
8. Huhta JC, Smallhorn JF, Macartney FJ, et al: Cross-sectional echocardiographic diagnosis of systemic venous return. Br Heart J 48:388-403, 1982.
9. Vick GW, Murphy DJ, Ludomirsky A, et al: Pulmonary venous and systemic ventricular inflow obstruction in patients with congenital heart disease: Detection by combined two-dimensional and Doppler echocardiography. J Am Coll Cardiol, 1986 (in press).
10. Huhta JC, Gutgesell HP, Nihill MR: Cross-sectional echocardiographic diagnosis of total anomalous pulmonary venous connection. Br Heart J 53:525-534, 1984.
11. Vitarelli A, Scapata A, Sanguigni V, Caminiti MC: Evaluation of total anomalous pulmonary venous drainage with cross-sectional colour-flow Doppler echocardiography. Eur Heart J 7:190-195, 1986.

Chapter 11

Fetal Examination

James C. Huhta, M.D.

Doppler echocardiography has rapidly found its way into the evaluation of the fetal cardiovascular system, including the measurement of intracardiac velocities at the atrioventricular and semilunar valves, detection of valve regurgitation, and assessment of placental function.[1-3] Because of its ability to provide spatial resolution to the pulsed Doppler study, color Doppler has the potential to facilitate the application of Doppler to the fetal examination. That is, it can quickly provide a technique for identifying the location and direction of blood flow velocities in structures identified by imaging.[4] In selected situations where imaging of the fetal heart is difficult, such as with polyhydramnios, oligohydramnios, and late gestational age, color Doppler may aid the pulsed Doppler examination. Imaging of flow velocities in the fetus in areas where two-dimensional imaging is of marginal quality allows placement of the pulsed Doppler sample volume in alignment with the jet even when the structure of interest is poorly seen. In many instances the optimal angle for imaging is orthogonal to the direction of blood flow. Standard echocardiographic examination in the fetus can be optimized for either imaging or Doppler, but not both. This technique, combining two-dimensional imaging and Doppler, therefore has obvious advantages.

Equipment Limitations

One difficulty of color Doppler in the fetus is the increased *depth* of the cardiac structures from the ultrasonic transducer and the limited peak repetition frequency leading to aliasing. In currently available equipment this velocity ambiguity at depth makes it difficult to know with certainty what the direction of blood flow is because of the possibility of multiple aliasing and reversal of direction coding. The highest velocity in the normal fetus is at the ductus arteriosus and ranges from 60 to 140 centimeters per second. Therefore, a depth of only 5 centimeters or more will produce aliasing of the "normal" velocity. However, in some fetuses oriented in an occiput posterior position and a posterior placenta, the normal velocities of blood flow in the fetus in the right ventricular outflow tract, for example, give an appearance similar to that found after birth (Figure 11-1). Therefore, the depth of the fetus limits what can be accomplished by color Doppler using current equipment.

Another reason for this is the limited *sensitivity* at depth of current technology. Above the frequency (velocity) cut-off of the machine there is a sensitivity below which no Doppler display will result or only noise will result from increasing the color display gain. This is dependent, in part, on the number of moving red blood cells reflecting ultrasound energy, as well as the usual Doppler angle considerations. Since the fetal ventricles eject less blood at velocities similar to those in neonates and children, the intensities are less and the problems of flow detection are compounded, placing further requirements on the equipment.

Another limitation of color Doppler technology in the fetal examination is the degraded *spatial resolution* during display of the velocity map. This is a function of the phased-array technology now used in most equipment with a maximum frequency of 5 MHz for imaging. Decreased *temporal resolution* due to the time necessary for the computation of the velocity map also leads to some degradation in imaging. This can be improved somewhat if a field of view narrower than a 90-degree sector is used. The application of mechanical annular array technology to this problem should allow optimized imaging at one frequency and color Doppler at another.

A fundamental concept of color Doppler is the *angle dependence* of flow velocity imaging and the impact of fetal position and image projection on what can be seen during any particular examination. The use of Doppler in the fetus for quantitation of blood flow velocity is limited because of the difficulty in aligning the pulsed Doppler sample volume axis with the instantaneous

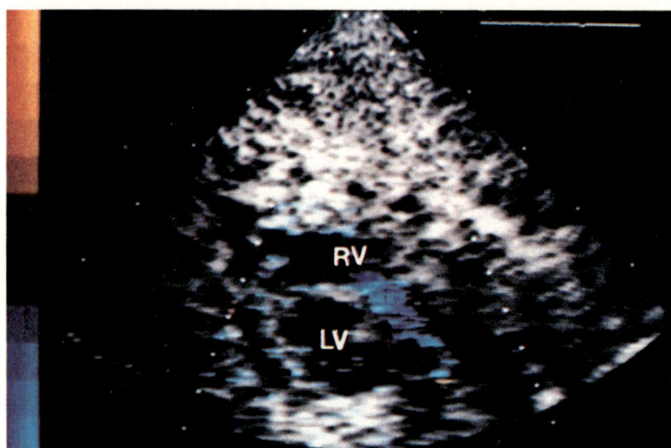

FIGURE 11-1—*Normal blood flow velocity in systole in the right ventricular outflow tract in a fetus of 26 weeks gestation. (Reproduced with permission from: Huhta JC: Uses and abuses of fetal echocardiography: A pediatric cardiologist's view. J Am Coll Cardiol 2:451-458, 1986.)*

three-dimensional blood flow column in axial, lateral, and azimuthal planes (Figure 11-2). The maximum velocity will be obtained when the angle with the direction of blood flow is zero in all three planes. Imaging adequate to visualize a structure in two dimensions plus the added information of flow velocity orientation and intensity make this process more accurate and readily achieved, but a persistent problem is measurement of the cross-sectional area of the flow in the tiny fetal heart. *Angle correction* is hazardous based only on the image of the structure of interest but may be more accurate when a color Doppler velocity map shows the direction of flow. Continuous-wave Doppler may also be used for the measurement of fetal blood flow velocities such as those in the ascending aorta (Figure 11-3).

At the present time, the resolution of the color velocity map is less than the best possible imaging available with the same transducer. In a way, these conflicting requirements—improved imaging resolution and better Doppler velocity characteristics—are at odds, the former requiring higher-frequency transducers and the latter lower. A color Doppler display optimized for the fetal examination may be possible by combining new technologies such as a hybridized annular array system or dual frequency dynamically focused phased-array imaging plus Doppler.

Safety

Pulsed Doppler intensities in the fetus may exceed the peak recommended levels expressed as spatial peak, peak average as recommended by the Food and Drug Administration. Color Doppler will, in general, have a

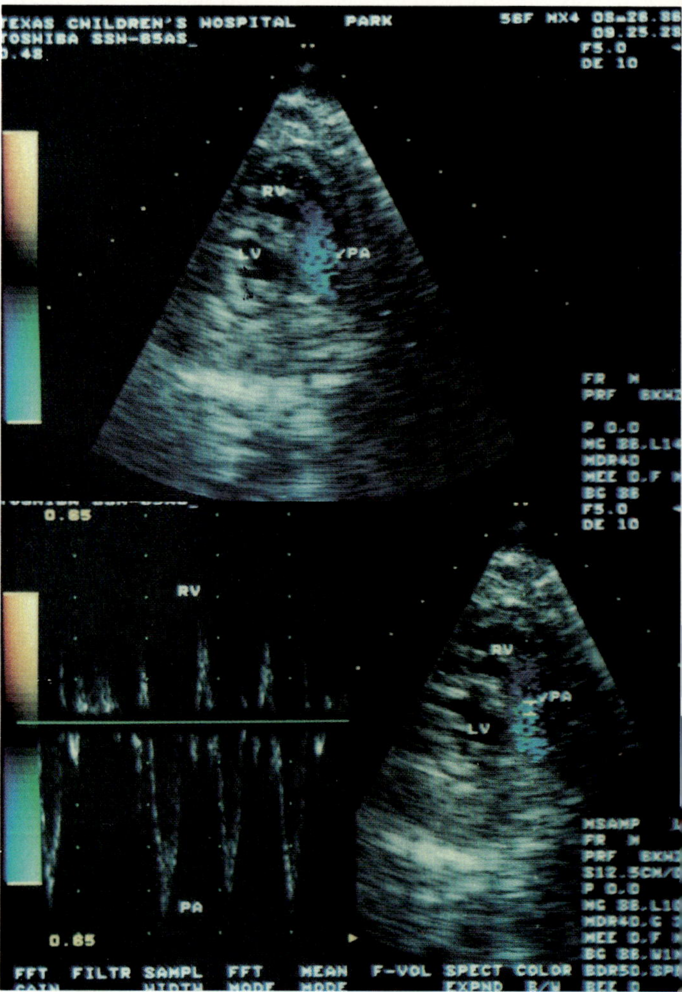

FIGURE 11-2—*Pulsed Doppler sampling in the pulmonary artery (PA) in a fetus, guided by color Doppler (blue color in systole). The pulsed Doppler sample volume was placed in the center of the color Doppler display (lower panel) and the resulting velocity was 50 centimeters per second. LV = left ventricle; RV = right ventricle.*

lower peak intensity than pulsed Doppler and may be safer from this point of view. As with all Doppler evaluation of the fetus, the intensity of the ultrasound energy must be minimized. We attempt to keep all Doppler intensities under the 100 milliwatt/cm^2 SPTA (spatial peak temporal average) level.

Some jets of blood flow velocity may be unmeasurable with pulsed Doppler techniques and *continuous-wave Doppler* may be necessary. Although the intensity is constant, the maximum level is less with continuous-wave techniques than with pulsed. In either situation, Doppler techniques should be used only when there is an indication of a problem or evidence that the Doppler information will add to the examination. We perform a cardiovascular examination of a fetus using ultrasound

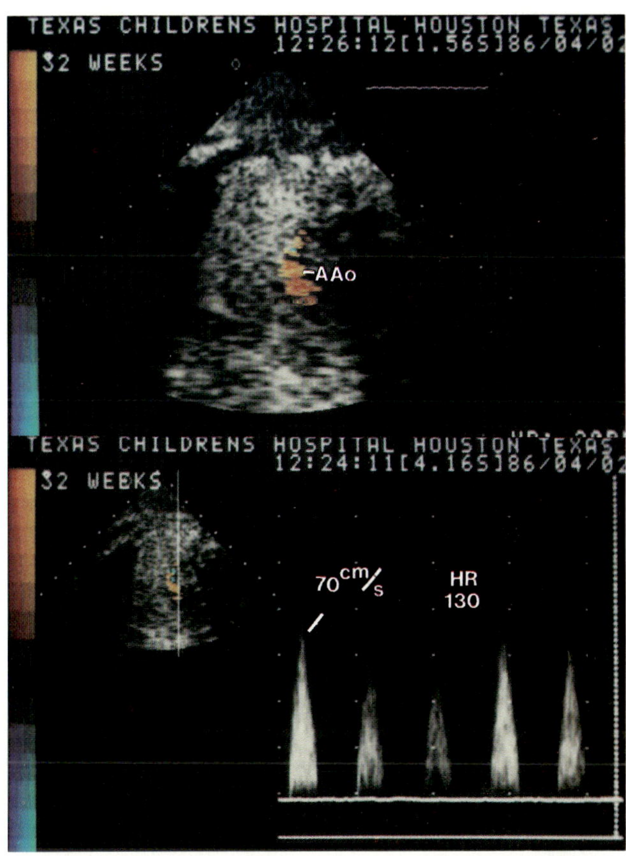

FIGURE 11-3—*Color Doppler in the ascending aorta (AAo) in a normal 32-week gestation fetus and the corresponding continuous-wave Doppler tracing (lower panel) with a peak systolic velocity of 70 centimeters per second.*

only when consulted by perinatal colleagues and when there is clear indication. We believe that Doppler evaluation of the heart goes hand in hand with the two-dimensional echocardiography examination and should be used in the fetus by those fully experienced with Doppler in the neonate and child. The intensities of *color Doppler* are somewhat less than routine pulsed Doppler at any one point in space so that the major concern about Doppler energy, that is, the possibility of high intensities at any one point, is less than with pulsed Doppler, whereas there is a more widespread field of exposure in this modality. During the test every effort should be made to avoid Doppler exposure to the fetal head.

The Normal Examination

Color Doppler allows visualization of the flow velocities in the developing heart. The flow of blood into the fetal ventricles in cardiac diastole will be coded as

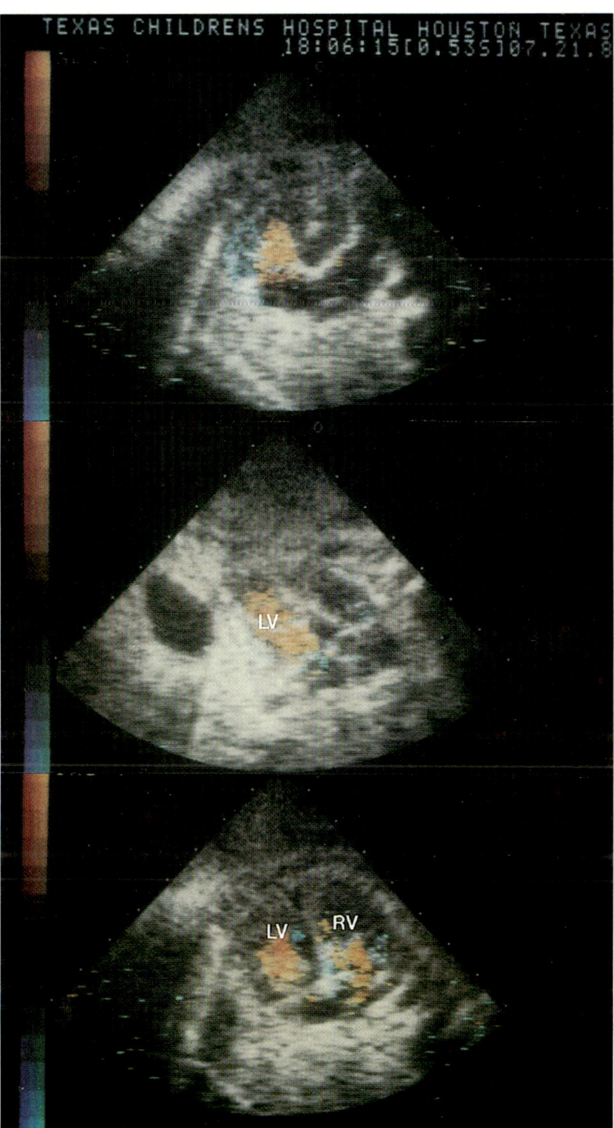

FIGURE 11-4—*Multiple color Doppler projections of normal filling of the left (LV) and right ventricles (RV) during a fetal examination. The diastolic filling is coded red or orange because the fetus is oriented so that the velocity is toward the transducer.*

a red or orange color when the apex of the fetal heart is toward the transducer (Figure 11-4). In this situation, the systolic velocities can be differentiated from the diastolic by the blue coding from blood flow velocity away from the transducer. The appearance of the jet may be an aid to the recognition of the source of the blood flow velocity. For example, the normal systolic velocities arising from the *ventricular outlets* are relatively narrow compared to diastolic velocities at the *atrioventricular valves*, and tend to cross with the ascending aorta flow passing superior and the pulmonary flow passing posterior and slightly inferior (Figure 11-5). The velocity in the main pulmonary artery accelerates toward the *ductus arteriosus* with frequent aliasing, depending on the angle (Figure 11-6). Flow in the aortic arch reverses direction and therefore will have opposite color coding in a systolic frame (Figure 11-7). Venous flows, particularly in the *inferior and superior vena cavae*, can be imaged and the pattern of flow intermixing in the right atrium can sometimes be appreciated with the inferior vena caval flow directed via the fossa ovalis (Figure 11-8) to the left atrium and the superior caval flow toward the tricuspid valve. In general, detection of flow velocity in the ductus venosus and the descending aorta is sporadic owing to the usual orientation of the fetus parallel to the imaging plane but orthogonal to the optimal Doppler orientation. The umbilical cord can be detected easily by imaging and color Doppler aids in differentiating the umbilical arteries and vein (see below).

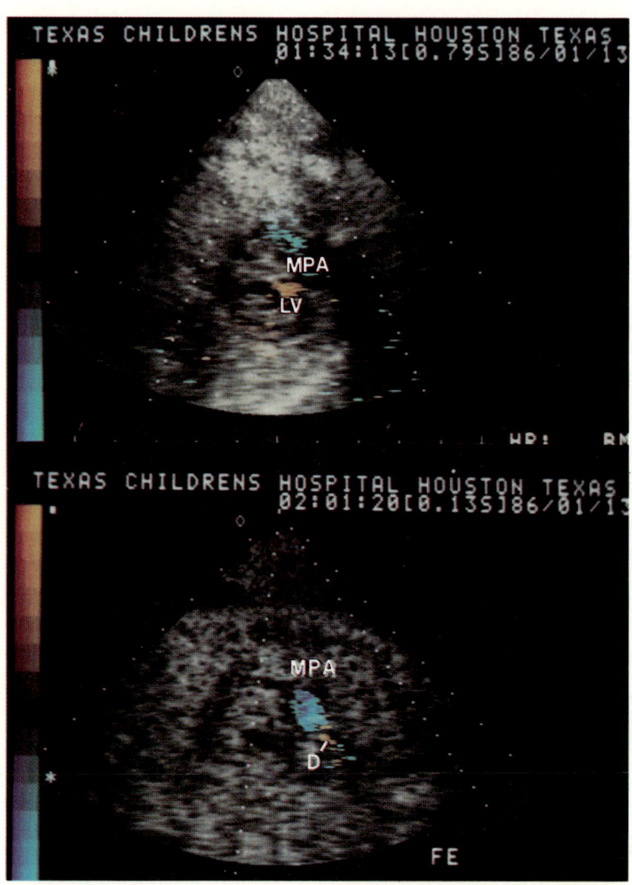

FIGURE 11-5—*Normal pulmonary (MPA) and ductal (D) color Doppler. The left ventricular outflow is oriented perpendicular and is coded red (upper panel).*

Valve Stenosis

Stenosis of a semilunar valve (aortic or pulmonary) may be difficult to detect in the fetus. Mild or moderately severe obstruction to ventricular ejection may not manifest as a significant abnormality of the valve or ventricle and the Doppler velocity may not be elevated because the pressure that the ventricle sees is already systemic in the fetus, and a ventricle-to-great-artery gradient would require normal ventricular function and normal ventricular output (no significant redistribution of blood flow). Even with severe semilunar valve stenosis and myocardial hypertrophy, early experience with pulsed Doppler has shown maximal velocities less than 2 meters per second corresponding to a peak systolic gradient of only 16 mmHg (gradient = $4\ V^2 = 4 \times 2^2 = 16$ mmHg).

Color Doppler may aid in the detection of valve stenosis if there is stenosis at a ventricular outlet and not atresia, and or in identifying the presence of increased flow in the other great artery, as is usually the case, e.g., large right ventricular stroke volume flow in aortic stenosis and large aortic flow in pulmonary stenosis with hypoplasia of the pulmonary arteries (Figure 11-9).

In complex types of congenital heart disease (see Chapter 6) such as tricuspid atresia, there may be hypoplasia of the right ventricle because of reduced flow through it and a ventricular septal defect (Figure 11-10). In such a situation, neither ventricular pressure can rise above that in the aorta and the presence of pulmonary stenosis at the valve may be difficult to detect (Figure 11-11). M-mode color Doppler may be useful to identify the source of the abnormal systolic velocity in a fetus. It has the advantage of improved temporal resolution. A

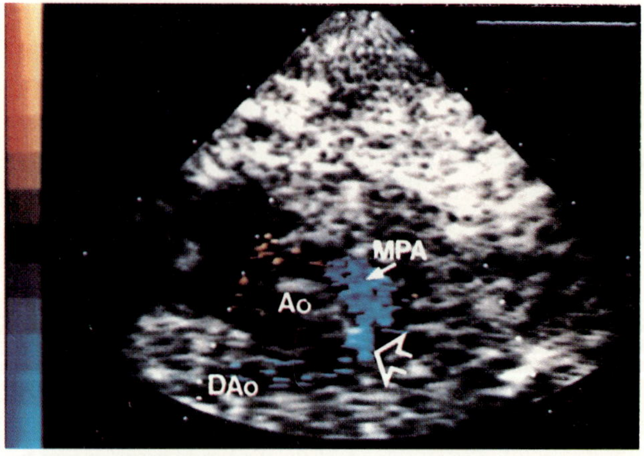

FIGURE 11-6—*Color Doppler in the normal fetal ductus arteriosus demonstrating aliasing (change of color from blue to green) in systole. (Reproduced with permission from: Huhta JC: Uses and abuses of fetal echocardiography: A pediatric cardiologist's view. J Am Coll Cardiol 2:451-458, 1986.)*

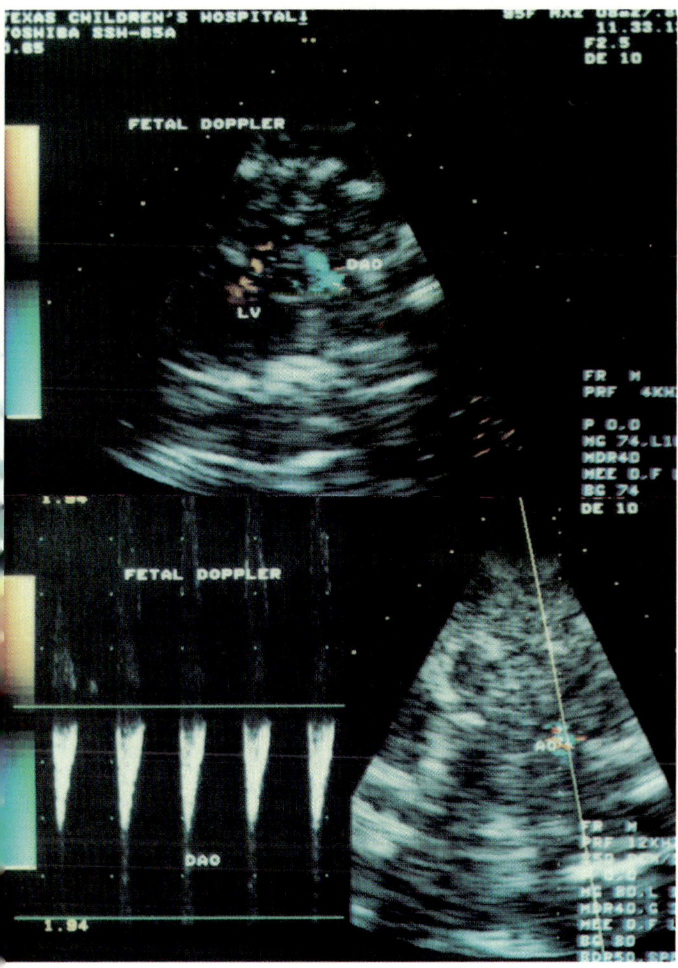

FIGURE 11-7—*Normal fetal aorta (orange) arising from the left ventricle (LV). The descending aorta (DAO) velocity by continuous-wave Doppler was 1.2 meters per second (lower panel). Note the color reversal from the ascending to descending aorta.*

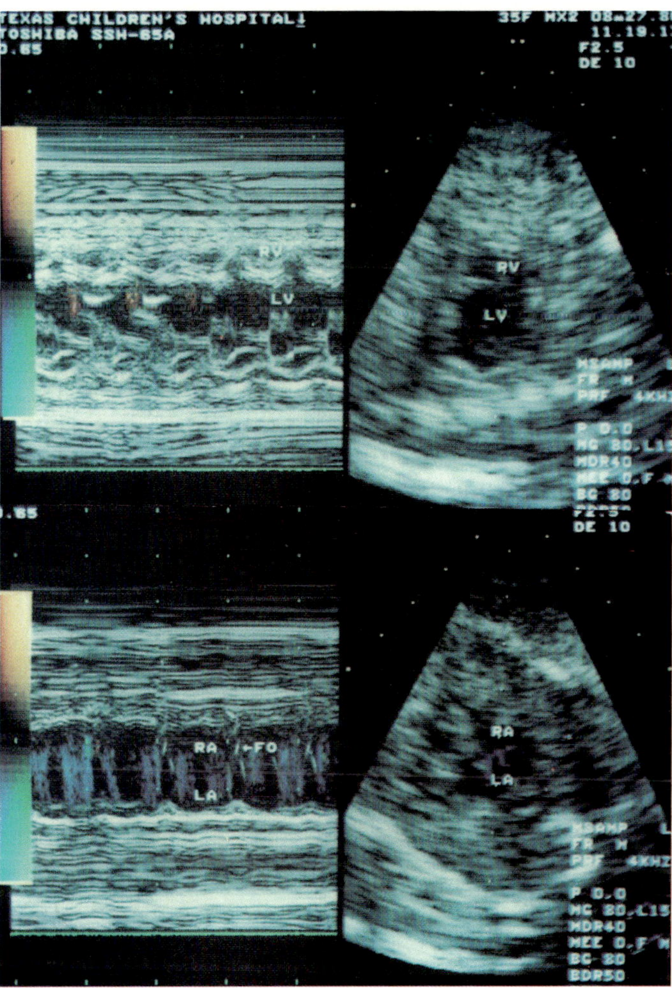

FIGURE 11-8—*Color Doppler with a M-mode display format in a 28-week gestation fetus with tricuspid atresia illustrating systolic ejection from the left ventricle (LV) (upper panel) and flow across the fossa ovalis (FO) away from the transducer (blue) from the right to left atrium (RA to LA) in the lower panel. RV = right ventricular outlet chamber.*

comparison of the systolic velocities in the descending aorta and the pulmonary artery in just such a fetus with tricuspid atresia and normally related great arteries and valvular pulmonary stensois showed a velocity of 1.6 meters per second downstream from the pulmonary valve and a descending aortic velocity of 1.0 meter per second (Figure 11-12).

Valve Insufficiency

Insufficiency or regurgitation of an atrioventricular or semilunar valve in the fetus, if severe, could lead to fetal demise from cardiac failure. Pulsed Doppler can be used for the diagnosis of tricuspid or mitral insufficiency,[6,7] and newer, more sensitive color Doppler equipment should allow more accurate assessment of this problem (see Chapter 4). Trivial degrees of tricuspid valve insufficiency are expected in utero and are common after birth in the neonatal period. But in association with hydrops fetalis, and congenital heart disease, valve insufficiency is an ominous sign and may indicate a form of congenital heart disease that is not passive before birth.[7] Color Doppler is needed in such a situation in order to assess not only the presence of regurgitation but its severity as well. At the present time there is no information available regarding this application of color Doppler.

Placental Assessment

Placental function assessment depends on aligning the Doppler sample volume with either the continuous

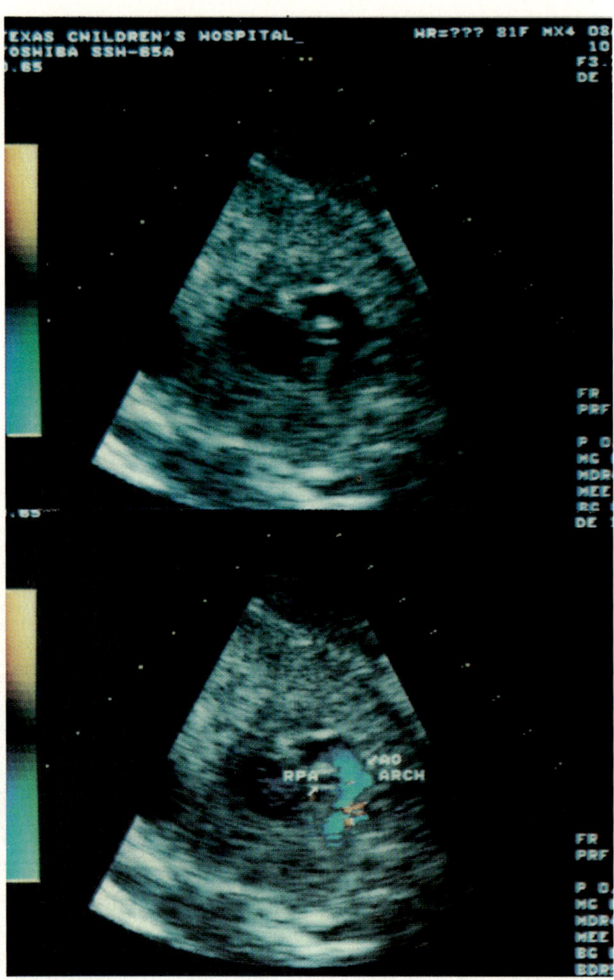

FIGURE 11-9—*Imaging (upper panel) and color Doppler (lower panel) of the aortic arch in the fetus described in Figure 11-8. Reduced pulmonary blood flow results in a prominent aortic arch (AO) and hypoplasia of the right pulmonary artery (RPA). Note the aliasing occurring in the descending aorta.*

or the pulsatile flow velocity map of the umbilical vein or artery respectively. Evaluation of the umbilical artery velocity wave form is being investigated as a method of assessing the flow to the placenta.[8,9] The pulsatility or systolic/diastolic velocity ratio correlates with the placental resistance with a higher ratio indicating a higher resistance (normal values after 32 weeks less than 3:1).

The course of the umbilical artery can be determined quickly using color Doppler to guide the placement of the pulsed Doppler sampling (Figure 11-13). With an anterior placenta, velocity in the artery will be coded orange and pulsatile. The umbilical venous flow velocity will be coded blue (away from the transducer).

As information analysis technology advances, the spinoffs for the ultrasound equipment industry and the applications of color Doppler display techniques to difficult diagnostic situations such as the cardiovascular assessment of the fetus will expand rapidly.

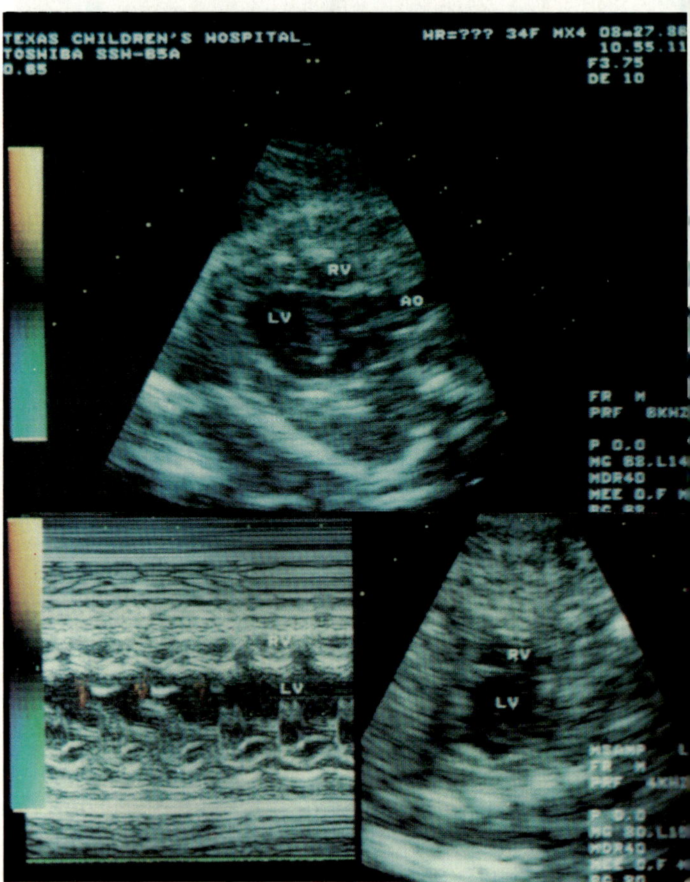

FIGURE 11-10—*Long- and short-axis views of a fetus with tricuspid atresia showing enlargement of the left ventricle (LV) and hypoplasia of the right ventricle (RV) and a normal LV outlet to the ascending aorta (AO). Higher short-axis scans show the ventricular septal defect between the LV and RV (lower panel).*

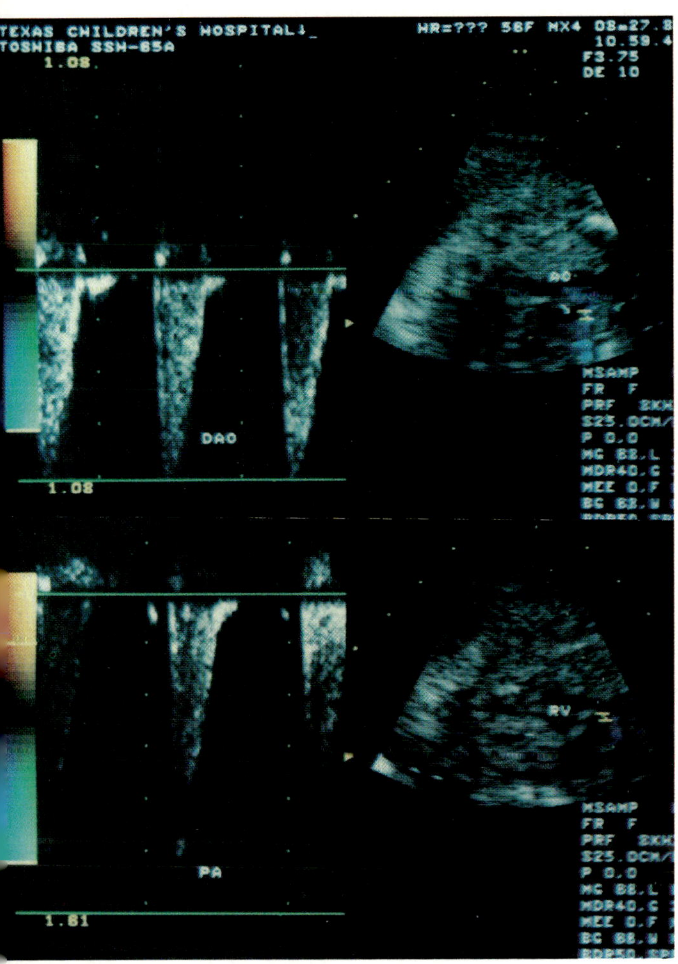

FIGURE 11-11—*Pulsed Doppler in the great arteries in a fetus with tricuspid atresia with normally related great arteries and pulmonary valve stenosis. Sampling in the descending aorta (DAO) (upper panel) shows a maximum velocity of 1.1 meters per second; however, the velocity in the pulmonary artery (PA) distal to the right ventricular outlet chamber (RV) was nearly 1.6 meters per second, which suggests RV outflow obstruction.*

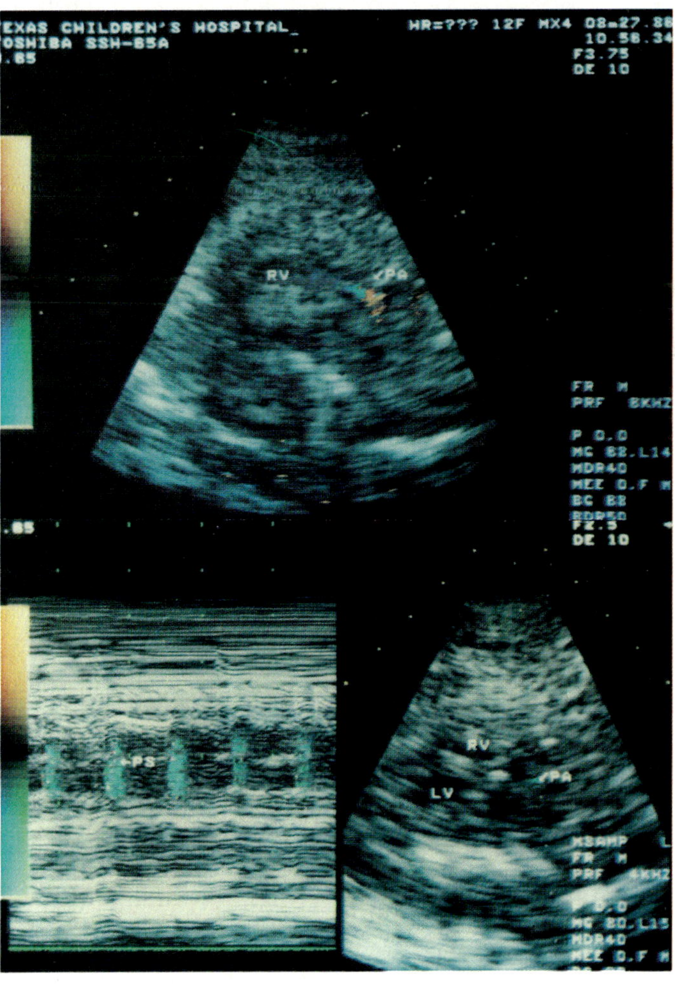

FIGURE 11-12—*Color Doppler of pulmonary valve stenosis with tricuspid atresia in a 28-week fetus showing aliasing in the pulmonary artery (PA) (upper panel) and color M-mode of the systolic turbulence in the pulmonary artery (PS, lower panel). RV = right ventricular outflow chamber.*

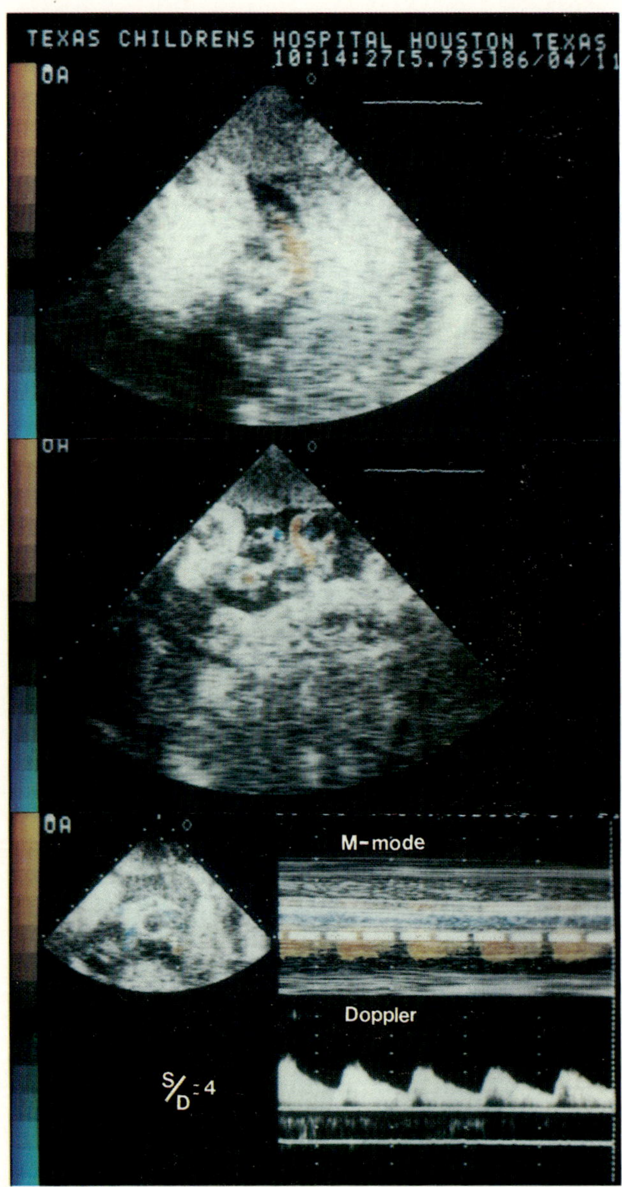

FIGURE 11-13—*Color Doppler in the umbilical cord showing phasic flow velocity toward the transducer coded orange in the umbilical artery (upper two panels). The color M-mode and pulsed Doppler displays (lower panel) show a systolic/diastolic (S/D) velocity ratio of 4 in this second-trimester normal fetus.*

References

1. Sahn DJ: Real-time 2-dimensional Doppler echocardiographic flow mapping. Circulation 71:849-853, 1985.
2. Huhta JC, Strasburger JF, Carpenter RJ, et al: Pulsed Doppler fetal echocardiography. J Clin Ultrasound 13:247-254, 1982.
3. Maulik D, Nanda NC, Saini VD: Fetal Doppler echocardiography: Methods and characterization of normal and abnormal hemodynamics. Am J Cardiol 53:572-578, 1984.
4. De Vore GR, Hornstein J, Siassi B, Platt LD: Doppler color flow mapping: Its use in the prenatal diagnosis of congenital heart disease in the human fetus. Echocardiography 2:551-557, 1985.
5. Friedman DM, Rutkowski M: Color flow mapping in the fetus: A new two-dimensional Doppler technique. J Card Ultrasonography 4:171-174, 1985.
6. Reiter AA, Huhta JC, Carpenter RJ, Klima T: Prenatal diagnosis of endocardial fibroelastosis in a monozygotic twin. J Cardiovasc Ultrasonography 4:225-228, 1985.
7. Silverman NH, Kleinman CS, Rudolph AM, et al: Fetal atrioventricular valve insufficiency associated with nonimmune hydrops: A two-dimensional echocardiographic and pulsed Doppler ultrasound study. Circulation 72:825-832, 1985.
8. Trudinger BJ, Giles WB, Cook CM, et al: Fetal umbilical artery flow velocity waveforms and placental resistance: Clinical significance. Br J Obstet Gynaecol 132:425-429, 1977.
9. Campbell S, Griffin DR, Pearce JM, et al: New Doppler technique for assessing uteroplacental blood flow. Lancet 1:675- 677, 1983.

Index